Livestock Economics for Students and Entrepreneurs

NIPA® GENX ELECTRONIC RESOURCES & SOLUTIONS P. LTD.
New Delhi-110 034

About the Author

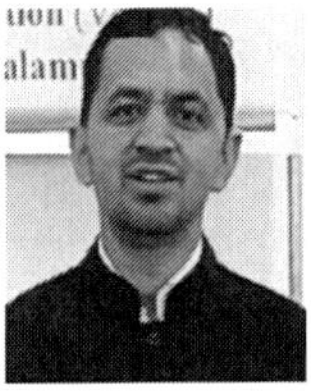

Dr. Devesh Thakur has been serving as a Faculty Member at the College of Veterinary and Animal Sciences, CSKHPKV Palampur, for over 16 years. He holds MVSC and PhD degrees from the prestigious Indian Veterinary Research Institute, where his academic excellence was highlighted by securing top rank in the Indian Council of Agricultural Research Postgraduate examination.

Specializing in **Veterinary Extension Education**, Dr. Thakur's postgraduate research explored the critical role of gender factors in dairy farming. His 16-year career is marked by significant contributions to education, research, and extension activities. He has an extensive publication record, including 74 research papers, 198 popular articles, 13 technical bulletins, and five books. His notable works include Gender Factor in Access to Livestock-based Information in India, Livestock Entrepreneurship, Dairy Entrepreneurship, Gender Perspectives in Animal Husbandry, Use of Social Media in Agriculture and Animal Husbandry. Additionally, he has developed a 10-hour Online Course with 86 videos on Public Speaking, Communications, and Interpersonal Skills, showcasing his innovative approach to education.

As a Principal Investigator, Dr. Thakur has led eleven action research projects funded by esteemed organizations such as NIF-DST India, NABARD, HIMCOSTE, National Commission of Women, and ICAR-IASRI, New Delhi. His grassroots engagement includes conducting numerous training programs, Model Training Programmes, and workshops for veterinarians, para-veterinary staff, extension officers, and farmers. These initiatives, supported by entities like the Agriculture Skill Council of India, National Commission of Women, Ministry of Agriculture (Government of India), NIFTEM, and ICAR, focus on practical aspects of Dairy, Sheep, Goat, and Poultry Farming.

Dr. Devesh Thakur's Livestock Economics for Students and Entrepreneurs offers a clear, industry-focused introduction to economics, tailored for the Veterinary Council of India (VCI) syllabus and aspiring animal husbandry entrepreneurs. Unlike traditional textbooks, it bridges complex theories with practical realities of dairy, poultry, and livestock management. With diverse question types, this comprehensive resource is essential for students, educators, researchers, and professionals.

Livestock Economics for Students and Entrepreneurs

Devesh Thakur
Assistant Professor
Department of Veterinary and AH Extension Education
DGCN College of Veterinary and Animal Sciences
Himachal Pradesh Agricultural University
Palampur, 176061, Himachal Pradesh

NIPA® GENX ELECTRONIC RESOURCES & SOLUTIONS P. LTD.
New Delhi-110 034

NIPA® GENX ELECTRONIC
RESOURCES & SOLUTIONS P. LTD.
101,103, Vikas Surya Plaza, CU Block
L.S.C. Market, Pitam Pura, New Delhi-110 034
Ph : +91-11-43860225, Mob.: +91 9717133558, 9540816132
E-mail: newindiapublishingagency@gmail.com
Website: www.nipaersources.com

Print ISBN: 978-93-58873-77-1
ebook ISBN: 978-93-58876-61-1

Composed and Designed by NIPA®.

Preface

For students and practitioners of veterinary science and animal husbandry, economics can often seem like an elusive subject, shrouded in complex theories and abstract models. Traditional economics textbooks, while rigorous, frequently fail to address the unique challenges and opportunities within the livestock sector, leaving learners disconnected from the practical realities of dairy farms, poultry operations, and livestock management. This book seeks to change that narrative, offering a clear, accessible, and industry-focused introduction to economics tailored specifically for the Veterinary Council of India (VCI) syllabus and aspiring entrepreneurs in animal husbandry.

This book comprehensively covers the foundational concepts of economics as outlined in the VCI curriculum, including demand and supply, utility, production theories, and factors of production. Each topic is presented with clarity and simplicity, ensuring that even those new to economics can grasp its principles with ease. What sets this book apart is its unwavering commitment to relevance: every concept is illustrated through vivid, real-world examples drawn from the dairy, livestock, and poultry industries. For instance, the law of demand is explored through the lens of milk pricing in rural markets, while the law of diminishing marginal utility is applied to optimizing feed allocation for cattle. These examples transform abstract ideas into practical tools for decision-making in animal husbandry.

To introduce deeper understanding and critical thinking, each chapter includes a set of analytical questions that challenge readers to apply economic principles to everyday scenarios in the livestock sector. Whether it's calculating the elasticity of demand for poultry products or analysing cost structures for a dairy cooperative, these questions bridge theory and practice, equipping students with the skills to tackle real-world challenges. Additionally, each chapter concludes with case studies based questions to build successful ventures in dairy, poultry, and livestock production.

This book is designed to serve multiple audiences. For veterinary students, it provides a clear and engaging roadmap to mastering the VCI syllabus, with practical insights that enhance academic success. For educators, it offers a wealth of teaching tools, including relatable examples and thought-provoking questions, to bring economics to life in the classroom. For prospective entrepreneurs, it serves as a guide to understanding the economic forces shaping the livestock sector, from market dynamics to cost management, empowering them to make informed business decisions.

In a world where the livestock industry plays a vital role in food security, rural livelihoods, and economic development, understanding economics is not just an academic exercise—it's a necessity. This book aims to empower its readers with the knowledge, skills, and inspiration to navigate the economic landscape of veterinary science and animal husbandry with confidence. Whether you're a student preparing for exams, an educator shaping the next generation, or an entrepreneur dreaming of a thriving livestock business, this book is your companion on the journey to economic fluency and success.

Contents

1

Introduction to Economics and Livestock Economics

Evolution of Economics as a Discipline

1. Initially, economics was not a separate subject but a part of **politics, ethics, and jurisprudence**.
2. The study of economic ideas gained prominence through discussions on wealth, trade, and resource management.
3. **Adam Smith's** book, *An Inquiry into the Nature and Causes of the Wealth of Nations* (1776), established economics as a distinct discipline.
4. Due to his contributions, Adam Smith is regarded as the **Father of Economics**.

Origin of the Term "Economics"

1. The word **Economics** is derived from the Greek term **"Oikonomikos"**:

   a) Oikos – Household

   b) Nomos – Management
2. Originally, **Oikonomikos** referred to the management of household affairs.

Scope of Economics

1. Economics studies **human activities related to wealth**—its production, distribution, and consumption.
2. Activities **not related to wealth** are generally considered outside the scope of economics.

Why Do We Study Economics?

1. Human wants are unlimited, but resources are limited.
2. Economics helps us understand **how individuals and societies make choices** regarding resource allocation to satisfy these unlimited wants.
3. The central issue in economics is **scarcity**—the gap between limited resources and unlimited human desires.

Definitions of Economics and Their Evolution

Economics has grown from a narrow focus on wealth to a broad study of human choices, resources, and growth. Each definition reflects its era's priorities and challenges

1. Wealth Definition – Adam Smith

1. Economics is the "science of wealth"—how it's produced, distributed, and grown. Adam Smith (1776, *The Wealth of Nations*) saw it as a study of what makes nations rich.
2. Example: For example wealth definition can explain that country like New Zealand has a highly efficient dairy and livestock industry. It produces more dairy products (like milk, cheese, and butter) than its population consumes. The surplus is exported to other countries, generating significant income

Critique

1. **Too Narrow:** Had a **narrow focus on wealth**, ignoring the **human and social aspects** of economics.
2. "**Dismal Science**" Label: Economics was labelled a **"dismal science"** because it emphasized **material wealth** over **social welfare**.
3. **Spiritual Pushback**: **Many philosophers** criticized this definition, influenced by **religious and spiritual values**, arguing that **mere wealth acquisition is not the ultimate goal of human activity.**
4. **Missed the Point:** Man's wants, not just wealth, drive economics—Smith overlooked the human angle.

2. Welfare Definition – Alfred Marshall

1. Marshall redefined economics as the **study of mankind in the ordinary business of life**—it examines that part of individual and social action which is most closely connected with the attainment and with the use of the material requisites of well-being.
2. To put simply here we study how people manage their everyday lives, especially when it comes to making decisions about money, resources, and material things they need to live well. It looks at how individuals and societies work to get and use the stuff that makes life better.
3. Example: Imagine you earn Rs 2,0000 monthly and must decide how to spend it. To meet your basic needs (material requisites of well-being), you allocate Rs 8000 for rent, Rs3000 for groceries, and Rs1000 for transportation. With Rs 8000 left, you choose whether to save, invest, or spend on leisure, reflecting how people use resources for a better life.

On a larger scale, governments make similar decisions, allocating budgets for healthcare, education, and infrastructure to improve societal well-being. This is how economics studies individual and social choices in managing resources efficiently.

Economics is the study of "mankind in the ordinary business of life"—how people and societies use material resources to improve well-being (from *Principles of Economics*, 1890). **Core Idea** Shift from wealth to welfare—economics is about everyday choices for a better life, not just piling up cash.

Critique

1. **Too Economic**: Overemphasized **economic activities**, neglecting **non-economic activities** like social and cultural factors.
2. **Ordinary Bias**: Economics also plays a role in **extraordinary times,** such as **war, disasters, and crises**, which were not covered in this definition.
3. **Material Focus**: Focused on **material requisites of wellbeing**, ignoring the non-material activities like services such as services offered by a veterinarian) which are equally important in economics

3. Scarcity Definition – Lionel Robbins

1. Economics is the **study of human behaviour as a relationship between ends and scarce means which have alternative uses.**
2. **Core idea**: Ends i.e. Human wants are **unlimited**, but means i.e. resources are **limited** and have **alternative uses and there is problem of choice**
3. This definition is broader than earlier wealth- and welfare-based views, as it includes decision-making and resource allocation, making it more applicable to real-world economic challenges.
4. Example: Human wants or **ends** include desires like owning a car, a house, education, or leisure. However, the resources or **means** to fulfill these wants—such as money, time, and raw materials—are **scarce**. Since these resources have **alternative uses**, individuals must choose how to allocate them wisely. For example, money can be spent on food, saved for the future, or used to buy clothes. In simple terms, economics studies how people make choices when their wants are unlimited, but resources are limited and can be used in different ways.

Critique

1. **Positive, Not Normative:** Treats economics as positive science ignoring the normative aspects of economics. Focuses on "what is" (choices), not "what should be" (fairness, ethics).
2. **No Growth:** The growth and development aspect of economy was ignored in the definition.
3. **Not Just Scarcity:** Not all economic problems arise from **scarcity**; **misuse or mismanagement** of resources can also create crises.

4. Growth Definition – Paul Samuelson & John Maynard Keynes

Paul Samuelson said that economics is the study of how **men and societies** choose, with or without money to employ scarce productive resources which could have alternative uses to produce various commodities over time and distribute them for consumption now and in future among various people and groups of society.

Key Points

1. **Scarce productive resources**: Resources like land, labour, capital, and raw materials are limited.
2. **Alternative uses**: These resources can be used in different ways. For example, land can be used to grow crops, build a factory, or set up a park.
3. **Production and distribution**: Economics studies how societies decide what to produce, how to produce it, and who gets to consume it—both now and in the future.
4. **With or without money**: Economic decisions can involve money (e.g., buying and selling goods) or non-monetary exchanges (e.g., barter systems or community sharing).

Example

1. Imagine a small village with limited resources. The villagers have a piece of land that could be used to grow wheat, build a school, or set up a small factory. The village panchayat must decide **what to produce**—whether to grow wheat for food, build a school for education, or establish a factory to create jobs. They also need to decide **how to distribute the benefits**—who gets the food, who can attend the school, or who gets employed at the factory. Since resources are **scarce and have alternative uses**, these decisions involve **trade-offs**, requiring the villagers to choose the most beneficial option for their community.

Keynes defined economics as "The study of administration of scarce resources and of the determinants of employment and income"

Example: Consider a country facing high unemployment: The government must decide how to use its limited resources to create jobs. For example:

i. Should it invest in infrastructure projects (like building roads) to create jobs?
ii. Should it provide subsidies to businesses to encourage hiring?
iii. Should it focus on education and training to improve skills for future employment?
iv. These decisions affect employment levels and income distribution in the economy.

Key Features

1. Acknowledges both **short-term and long-term economic decisions**.
2. Considers **economic policies, technological advancements, and social structures** that impact economic growth.
3. Example: A **farmer investing in quality cattle feed** improves milk yield and income over time.

Conclusion

Each definition has shaped the way economics is studied today.

1. **Adam Smith** focused on **wealth**.
2. **Alfred Marshall** emphasized **welfare**.
3. **Lionel Robbins** defined economics as **scarcity and choice**.
4. **Samuelson & Keynes** broadened it to include **growth and development**.

Thus, modern economics is a dynamic field, integrating aspects of wealth, welfare, scarcity, and growth to address real-world challenges.

Additional Snippets

Economics has evolved

1. **Smith (Wealth):** "How do we get rich?".
2. **Marshall (Welfare):** "How do we live better?"
3. **Robbins (Scarcity):** "How do we choose with limits?"
4. **Samuelson & Keynes (Growth):** "How do we grow and share over time?"

Modern Economics

Blends all four—wealth (exports), welfare (living standards), scarcity (choices), and growth (jobs, tech). For vets and farmers, it's about balancing today's feed costs with tomorrow's milk profits.

Why the definitions matters for animal husbandry entrepreneur?

1. **Smith definition:** Track how your milk sales build wealth.
2. **Marshall definition**: Budget for cow care and family well-being.
3. **Robbins definition:** Choose between vet visits or new equipment.
4. **Samuelson & Keynes definition:** Invest in tech or training for long-term farm growth.

Key Takeaways

1. **Wealth:** Economics started with riches—good for trade stats.
2. **Welfare:** Shifted to life's quality—daily farm decisions.
3. **Scarcity:** Focused on choices—your Rs 50,000 dilemma.
4. **Growth:** Added time and jobs—future-proofing your herd.

5. Livestock Economics

Livestock Economics is the study of how people—within a country or across different nations-utilize scarce resources to produce livestock and their products in a manner that ensures the best advantage for mankind, both in the present and the future. It encompasses the efficient allocation of resources such as land, labor, capital, and technology to ensure the sustainable development of the livestock sector.

The ultimate goal is to achieve the **best advantage of mankind**, which includes a wide range of economic, social, and environmental objectives.

Best Advantages of Mankind through Livestock Production

1. Meeting Food Requirements

1. Livestock provides **essential nutrients** through products like **milk, meat, fat, and eggs**.
2. These are vital sources of **protein, vitamins, and minerals**, contributing to **food security** and improved public health.

2. Providing Sustainable Employment

1. The livestock sector creates **direct employment** for farmers, veterinarians, and workers in dairy, poultry, and meat processing industries.
2. It also supports **indirect employment** in feed production, transport, marketing, and veterinary services.

3. Providing Stable Income

1. Livestock farming ensures **regular earnings** through daily sales of **milk, eggs, and meat**.
2. It serves as an economic buffer, particularly in **rural areas**, where crop farming income may be seasonal.

4. Maintenance of Ecological Balance

1. Livestock contributes to **organic farming** through manure, reducing the need for chemical fertilizers.
2. Grazing animals help maintain **grassland ecosystems** and promote soil fertility.
3. Proper livestock management can aid in **carbon sequestration**, reducing environmental degradation.

5. Maintenance of Human-Animal Bond & Sentimental Values

1. In many cultures, livestock holds **religious, traditional, and emotional** significance.
2. Animals such as cows, buffaloes, and camels are **revered** and often protected beyond their economic utility.

6. Efficient Conversion of Non-Edible Crop Residues into Edible Products

1. Livestock helps in **waste utilization** by converting **crop residues, kitchen waste, and agro-industrial by-products** into high-value animal products.
2. Ruminants like cattle and sheep **digest fibrous feeds**, producing milk and meat from otherwise unusable resources.

Best Advantages of Mankind through Livestock Production: Some Examples

Livestock isn't just about profit—it delivers a bundle of benefits. Here's how:

1. Meeting Food Requirements

- **What It Does:** Supplies essentials like protein, vitamins, and minerals through milk, meat, fat, and eggs.
- **Impact:** Boosts food security and health—think kids growing strong on milk or adults fuelled by meat.

- **Example**
  - A dairy farm produces 1,000 litres of milk daily, rich in calcium and protein, feeding a village and cutting malnutrition.
  - Poultry farms churn out 10,000 eggs/week—affordable protein for urban families.

2. Providing Sustainable Employment

- **What It Does:** Creates jobs—direct (farmers, vets) and indirect (feed makers, truckers).
- **Impact:** Keeps rural economies alive and supports urban industries.
- **Example**
  - A goat farm employs 5 locals to milk and shear, plus a vet for check-ups.
  - Feed mills hire 20 workers to process maize for that farm—jobs ripple out.
  - **Dairy Co-op:** 50 farmers, 10 milk collectors, 2 vet, and 20 factory workers process 2,000L/day—82 jobs from 500 cows.

3. Providing Stable Income

- **What It Does:** Offers steady cash flow from daily/weekly sales, unlike seasonal crops.
- **Impact:** Acts as a financial safety net, especially in rural areas.
- **Example**
  - A dairy farmer earns Rs 3,000/day selling 50 liters of milk at Rs 60/liter—reliable income vs. waiting for a rice harvest.
  - A poultry farmer sells 500 eggs/week at Rs 10 each—Rs 5000 weekly cushions crop failures.

4. Maintenance of Ecological Balance

- **What It Does:** Supports green farming and ecosystems via manure and grazing.
- **Impact:** Cuts chemical use, boosts soil, and can trap carbon.
- **Example**
  - Cow manure fertilizes 10 acres organically, saving Rs 10,000/year on synthetic fertilizers.
  - Sheep grazing on 50 acres prevents overgrowth, keeps grasslands healthy, and sequesters carbon.

5. Maintenance of Human-Animal Bond & Sentimental Values

- **What It Does:** Honours cultural and emotional ties to animals.
- **Impact:** Preserves traditions and mental well-being beyond economics.
- **Example**
  - In India, cows are sacred—farmers keep them even if milk yield drops, valuing their spiritual role.
  - A camel herder in Rajasthan treasures his herd for heritage, not just meat or transport.
  - **Temple Cows:** A farmer keeps 5 old cows (low milk) for religious offerings—sells ghee at Rs 600/kg to devotees, blending faith and profit.

6. Efficient Conversion of Non-Edible Crop Residues into Edible Products

- **What It Does:** Turns waste (crop stalks, kitchen scraps) into food via livestock.
- **Impact:** Reduces waste, boosts efficiency—ruminants are nature's recyclers.
- **Example**
  - Cattle eat maize stalks after harvest, producing 5L milk/day per cow—food from "trash."
  - Sheep turn wheat straw into 2 kg meat/head—edible value from inedible stuff.

Key Areas of Study in Livestock Economics

1. **Resource Allocation**: How scarce resources like land, labor, and capital are allocated to livestock production.
2. **Production Efficiency**: Maximizing output (milk, meat, eggs) while minimizing input costs (feed, labor, medicines).
3. **Market Dynamics**: Understanding demand and supply, price determination, and trade of livestock products.
4. **Policy Analysis**: Evaluating the impact of government policies, subsidies, and regulations on the livestock sector.
5. **Sustainability**: Ensuring that livestock production meets present needs without compromising the ability of future generations to meet theirs.
6. **Risk Management**: Addressing risks such as disease outbreaks, climate change, and market fluctuations.

"A skilled vet can save an animal's life, but a vet who understands economics can save an entire farm."

Veterinarians and farmers who understand economics make **more informed, profitable, and sustainable** decisions. From pricing services to managing farm finances, mastering economics is key to success in modern animal agriculture.

Analytical Questions and Answers

Question 1

Define economics and explain how its definitions have evolved over time

Answer

Economics is the study of how individuals and societies allocate limited resources to satisfy unlimited human wants. It involves decision-making related to production, distribution, and consumption of goods and services.

The definitions of economics have evolved over time:

- **Adam Smith (Wealth Definition)** focused on the production and accumulation of wealth, calling economics the "science of wealth."
- **Alfred Marshall (Welfare Definition)** shifted the focus to human well-being, defining economics as the study of mankind in the ordinary business of life.
- **Lionel Robbins (Scarcity Definition)** emphasized the allocation of scarce resources among competing ends, introducing the concept of choice.
- **Samuelson and Keynes (Growth Definition)** expanded economics to include growth, resource allocation over time, and distribution with or without money.

This evolution reflects the changing priorities of societies—from wealth accumulation to welfare, decision-making, and sustainable growth.

Question 2

Explain the importance of studying economics in the field of animal husbandry

Answer

Studying economics is essential in animal husbandry because it helps stakeholders—farmers, veterinarians, policymakers—make informed decisions regarding the use of scarce resources.

Importance includes:

- **Efficient resource use:** Understanding costs and benefits in livestock feeding, breeding, and healthcare.

- **Profitability analysis:** Helps in calculating returns on investments like improved sheds or high-yielding animals.
- **Market understanding:** Economics aids in price setting, forecasting demand for milk, eggs, meat, etc.
- **Policy planning:** Economic analysis supports decisions on subsidies, insurance schemes, and rural employment.
- **Sustainability:** Guides balanced use of land, labor, and capital for long-term livestock sector growth.

Thus, economics helps maximize output, income, and social welfare in animal husbandry.

Question 3

Compare and contrast the definitions of economics given by Adam Smith, Alfred Marshall, and Lionel Robbins.

Answer

Feature	Adam Smith (Wealth)	Alfred Marshall (Welfare)	Lionel Robbins (Scarcity)
Focus	Wealth creation and accumulation	Human welfare and well-being	Scarcity, choice, and alternative uses
Viewpoint	Materialistic	Human-centric	Neutral and analytical
Scope	Narrow (only wealth-related activities)	Wider (material welfare of people)	Widest (all human behavior under scarcity)
Limitations	Ignores non-material aspects	Ignores extraordinary events, non-material gains	Ignores normative economics and growth aspects

Each definition reflects a stage in the development of economics: from wealth to welfare to rational decision-making under scarcity.

Question 4

How does livestock economics help in achieving the best advantage for mankind?

Answer

Livestock economics facilitates optimal utilization of resources in animal husbandry to improve human lives. It contributes to:

1. **Food security:** Provides milk, meat, eggs rich in protein and nutrients.
2. **Sustainable employment:** Creates jobs in production, processing, and support services.
3. **Stable income:** Ensures regular earnings from daily produce.

4. **Ecological balance:** Manure supports organic farming and grazing maintains soil health.
5. **Cultural and emotional values:** Strengthens human-animal bonds and respects traditional roles of livestock.
6. **Waste to wealth:** Converts non-edible crop residues into valuable food products.

Thus, livestock economics balances economic, social, and environmental goals for present and future generations.

Question 5

Discuss the scope of economics and why it is essential to study it.

Answer

The **scope of economics** includes the study of human activities related to:

- **Production:** Creating goods/services like milk or eggs.
- **Distribution:** Ensuring equitable access to resources and products.
- **Consumption:** Understanding how consumers utilize goods for satisfaction.

Non-economic activities such as religious or voluntary work are usually excluded.

Importance of studying economics

- Resources are **limited**, but human wants are **unlimited**.
- Economics helps us make **wise choices** in using these resources.
- It aids in planning, budgeting, and long-term **growth**.
- Essential for individuals, businesses, and governments to tackle **scarcity**, make investments, and ensure **welfare**.

In animal husbandry, economics supports decision-making in feed allocation, animal care, and marketing, ensuring both profitability and sustainability.

Question 6

Give suitable examples of how the four major definitions of economics are applied in livestock-based entrepreneurship.

Answer

- **Adam Smith (Wealth):** A dairy farmer tracks milk sales and expands his herd to increase wealth through surplus production and trade.
- **Alfred Marshall (Welfare):** A farmer budgets for both animal feed and children's education to enhance family well-being.

- **Lionel Robbins (Scarcity):** A farmer must choose whether to buy a milking machine or invest in veterinary services due to limited funds.
- **Samuelson/Keynes (Growth):** A poultry entrepreneur invests in training workers and modernizing equipment to boost long-term productivity and income.

These examples show how economics shapes everyday choices in livestock ventures.

Question 7

How can Adam Smith's Wealth Definition of economics be applied to improve the profitability of a dairy farm?

Answer

Adam Smith's Wealth Definition focuses on the production, distribution, and growth of wealth. For a dairy farm, this means maximizing milk production (output), optimizing distribution (selling to local markets or exporters), and increasing wealth over time (reinvesting profits). For example, a dairy farmer could adopt Smith's ideas by investing in high-yield cow breeds to boost milk production, negotiating export contracts like New Zealand's dairy industry (as mentioned in the chapter), and reinvesting earnings into better feed or equipment. This approach emphasizes efficiency and trade to build wealth, aligning with Smith's view. However, it might overlook cow welfare or environmental costs, which later definitions address.

Question 8

Using Alfred Marshall's Welfare Definition, how should a veterinarian prioritize budget allocation for a livestock farm facing financial constraints?

Answer

Marshall's Welfare Definition emphasizes using resources to improve well-being in everyday life. For a veterinarian managing a farm's budget (e.g., Rs 20,000/month), this means prioritizing spending on material requisites that enhance animal and farmer welfare—like health, productivity, and basic needs. For instance, allocating Rs 8,000 for vaccinations and medicines ensures cow health (vital for milk yield), Rs 5,000 for quality feed supports nutrition, and Rs 3,000 for basic farm upkeep maintains operations—all directly tied to well-being. The remaining Rs 4,000 could go to farmer training or savings, improving long-term welfare. Unlike Smith's wealth focus, Marshall's lens ensures decisions balance productivity with quality of life, though it might undervalue non-material factors like farmer morale or cultural practices (e.g., keeping sacred cows).

Question 9

How does Lionel Robbins' Scarcity Definition explain the trade-offs a poultry farmer faces when deciding between investing in feed or veterinary care?

Answer

Robbins defines economics as the study of human behavior in allocating scarce means (resources) with alternative uses to meet unlimited ends (wants). For a poultry farmer with a limited budget (e.g., Rs 10,000), the "scarce means" are money and time, while the "ends" include healthy chickens, high egg output, and profit. Investing Rs 7,000 in quality feed could boost egg production (e.g., 500 eggs/week at Rs 10 each = Rs 5,000), but skimping on veterinary care (Rs 3,000) risks disease outbreaks, wiping out the flock. Alternatively, spending Rs 7,000 on vet services ensures flock health but might reduce feed quality, lowering egg yield. Robbins' framework highlights this choice: resources are limited, and each option has trade-offs. The farmer must weigh short-term gains (feed) against long-term stability (health), reflecting scarcity-driven decision-making.

Question 10

How can Paul Samuelson's Growth Definition guide a goat farmer in planning for future expansion while managing current resources?

Answer

Samuelson's Growth Definition focuses on using scarce resources over time to produce and distribute goods for current and future consumption. For a goat farmer with 50 goats and limited land, this means balancing today's milk/meat output with tomorrow's herd growth. For example, the farmer could use land to grow fodder now (producing 100 liters of milk monthly, sold at Rs 50/liter = Rs 5,000) while reserving Rs 2,000 to buy two new goats, increasing the herd to 52. Over time, this expands production capacity (e.g., 104 liters/month in a year). The "alternative uses" of land—fodder vs. cash crops—require a choice: short-term income or long-term growth. Samuelson's lens encourages reinvestment and planning, ensuring the farm grows sustainably while meeting present needs, unlike Robbins' static scarcity focus.

Question 11

In the context of Keynes' emphasis on employment and income, how might a government policy supporting dairy cooperatives impact rural veterinarians and farmers?

Answer

Keynes' definition highlights managing scarce resources to boost employment and income. A government policy subsidizing dairy cooperatives (e.g., Rs 10/liter milk price support) could increase farmers' income, stabilizing rural economies. For example, a cooperative with 50 farmers producing 2,000 liters daily earns Rs 120,000/day (at Rs 60/liter market price + Rs 10 subsidy). This extra income could fund hiring two veterinarians (Rs 20,000/month each) to manage cow health, creating jobs and improving milk yields (e.g., from 4L to 5L/cow/day). The ripple effect—more milk, more income, more employment—aligns with Keynes' focus on resource administration for economic activity. However, if subsidies distort markets (e.g., overproduction), vets and farmers might face price drops, highlighting the need for balanced policy.

Question 12

How does livestock economics' focus on ecological balance influence a sheep farmer's decision to expand grazing land?

Answer

Livestock economics aims to optimize resource use for mankind's advantage, including ecological balance. A sheep farmer with 50 sheep grazing 50 acres might consider expanding to 75 acres to increase meat production (e.g., 2 kg/sheep = 100 kg to 150 kg total). However, overgrazing could degrade soil, reduce grass regrowth, and disrupt carbon sequestration, harming long-term sustainability.

Economically, maintaining 50 acres with rotational grazing might yield less meat now (100 kg at Rs 500/kg = Rs 50,000) but preserve soil fertility, ensuring future output.

Question 13

Why might a veterinarian recommend investing in waste-to-feed conversion systems, using the "efficient conversion of non-edible residues" advantage from livestock economics?

Answer

Livestock economics values converting non-edible crop residues into edible products, enhancing efficiency. A veterinarian might recommend a waste-to-feed system (e.g., silage from maize stalks) for a dairy farm because it cuts feed costs (e.g., from Rs 20/kg to Rs 5/kg using waste) while maintaining milk output (5L/cow/day at Rs 60/liter = Rs 300/cow/day). For 10 cows, this saves Rs 1,500/day on feed, boosting profit. Health-wise, properly processed residues prevent digestive issues, aligning with vet expertise. This leverages scarce resources (waste) for production, supports sustainability, and ties to Samuelson's growth focus—using innovation for long-term gains while meeting current needs.

Question 14

How can the "human-animal bond" advantage in livestock economics affect a farmer's decision to keep unproductive cows, and what economic trade-offs are involved?

Answer

The human-animal bond, a cultural advantage in livestock economics, values animals beyond profit—like sacred cows in India. A farmer with five old cows yielding just 1L/day each (vs. 5L for younger cows) might keep them for sentimental or religious reasons, selling ghee at Rs 600/kg to temples (5L milk = 0.5 kg ghee = Rs 300/day). Economically, replacing them with young cows could yield 25L/day (Rs 1,500/day), a Rs 1,200 daily loss. The trade-off pits welfare (Marshall's well-being) and tradition against wealth (Smith's focus). Livestock economics recognizes this non-monetary value, but the farmer must balance it with financial viability, perhaps offsetting costs by diversifying income (e.g., manure sales).

Question 15.

Compare and contrast the definitions of economics given by Adam Smith, Alfred Marshall, and Lionel Robbins, Paul Samuelson & J.M. Keynes (20th century)

Economist	Definition Focus	Key Elements	Merits	Limitations
Adam Smith (1776)	**Wealth Definition**	Economics is the science of wealth. Focuses on production and accumulation of wealth.	Pioneer of economics; emp hasized economic growth and trade.	Narrow and materialistic; ignored human welfare and social aspects.
Alfred Marshall (1890)	**Welfare Definition**	Economics is the study of mankind in the ordinary business of life. Concerned with material welfare.	Shifted focus to human well-being; included social relevance.	Ignores non-material aspects; ex cludes non-eco nomic behavior like charity.
Lionel Robbins (1932)	**Scarcity and Choice Definition**	Economics is a science of scarcity, choice, and alternative uses of resources.	Universally applicable; focuses on decision- making.	Too abstract; ignores welfare and moral values.
Paul Sam uelson & J.M. Keynes (20th century)	**Growth-Oriented Definition**	Economics is about allocating scarce resour ces over time for growth, stability, and development.	Dynamic and future-oriented; includes welfare, policy, and macro economics.	Broad and complex; difficult to apply in micro-level decisions.

2

Economics Explored Traditional and Modern Approaches Positive and Normative Perspectives

Approaches to study subject matter of economics

There are two approaches to study subject matter of economics-

1. **Traditional Approach**
2. **Modern Approach**

Economics studies human economic activities, which involve the creation, use, exchange, and distribution of wealth.

1. Traditional Approach

This approach splits economic activities into four interconnected areas: **Consumption, Production, Exchange, and Distribution (CPED).**

1. Consumption – Using Goods & Services

Consumption refers to the utilization of goods and services to satisfy human needs and wants. It involves the destruction of utility, meaning that once a good or service is consumed, it cannot be reused in its original form i.e. once used, their original form is gone (utility destroyed) Economics studies the nature of human wants, their characteristics, and how individuals make consumption decisions.

Examples in Animal Husbandry and Veterinary Care

- **Milk and Eggs:** A family drinks 5L milk/week (Rs 50/L) and eats 20 eggs (Rs 5 each)—protein and calcium needs met, utility gone after eating.
- **Vet Check-Up:** A farmer pays Rs 500 for a cow vaccination—health service consumed, cow protected, utility used up.
- **Fodder for Cows:** 50 kg fodder/week (Rs 10/kg) boosts milk yield—consumed by cows, not reusable, but drives production.

Key Insight

Consumption is the endgame—farmers and vets produce so people (and animals) can consume.

2. Production – Creation of Goods & Services

Production transforms resources into useful goods and services, thereby creating utility. It requires the coordination of four key factors of production:

1. **Land**: Natural resources: grazing land, water, and climate conditions.
2. **Labour**: Human effort (human sweat): farmers, veterinarians, and farm workers.
3. **Capital**: Investments in machinery, equipment, fodder, medicines, and infrastructure.
4. **Organisation (Entrepreneurship)**: Decision-making and management of resources to ensure efficient production.

Examples in Dairy and Veterinary Sectors

- **Milk Production**
  - i. Land: 10 acres for grazing.
  - ii. Labor: 2 workers milk 20 cows.
  - iii. Capital: Rs 50,000 milking machine.
  - iv. Organization: Farmer schedules milking, feeding—500L/week at Rs 50/L.
- **Eggs from Poultry**
  - i. Land: 1 acre area for poultry farm.
  - ii. Labor: 3 workers feed 1,000 hens.
  - iii. Capital: Rs 20,000 feed stock.
  - iv. Organization: Owner times egg collection—700 eggs/day, Rs 5 each.
- **Vet Services**
  - i. Land: Clinic space.
  - ii. Labor: Vet's expertise.
  - iii. Capital: Rs 10,000 ultrasound tool.
  - iv. Organization: Vet manages appointments—20 visits/week, Rs 500 each.

3. Exchange – Buying & Selling of Goods & Services

Exchange refers to the transfer of ownership of goods and services, which creats higher utility through legal and ethical means between individuals/regions/

countries etc. It facilitates the flow of goods and services from producers to consumers and can occur at various levels:

i. **Between individuals**: A farmer selling milk directly to a consumer.

ii. **Among regions and countries**: Export of dairy products like cheese, butter, or powdered milk.

iii. **Through markets**: Milk cooperatives, veterinary pharmacies, or online platforms for pet services.

Historically, the barter system was used, where goods were exchanged for other goods. Today, money serves as the medium of exchange, making transactions more efficient and scalable.

Examples in Animal Husbandry

i. A dairy farmer selling milk to a cooperative society or a private dairy company.

ii. A veterinary pharmacy selling medicines and supplements to livestock owners.

iii. An online platform facilitating the sale of organic milk, eggs, or poultry products.

4. Distribution – Sharing of Earnings

Distribution refers to how the income generated from production is allocated (divided) among the factors of production. It is also known as the theory of factor pricing, as each factor earns according to its contribution. It also refers sharing of utility.

Example of Distribution in a Dairy Farm

i. **Landowner**: Earns rent for providing land for cattle grazing or fodder cultivation.

ii. **Investor (Capitalist)**: Earns interest on capital invested in machinery, sheds, and equipment.

iii. **Workers**: Earn wages for tasks like milking, feeding, and caring for animals.

iv. **Entrepreneur (Dairy Farm Owner)**: Earns profit for managing production, sales, and overall operations.

Example of a Vet Clinic

i. **Land:** Rs 8,000 rent for clinic space.

ii. **Capital:** Rs 2,000 interest on Rs 50,000 equipment loan.

iii. **Labor:** Vet earns Rs 30,000 for 60 visits (Rs 500 each).

iv. **Organization:** Clinic owner pockets Rs 10,000 profit after costs.

2. Modern approach

The **modern view of economics** is broadly divided into two main branches: **Microeconomics** and **Macroeconomics proposed by Ragnar Frisch**. Each branch focuses on different aspects of economic activity and provides unique insights into how economies function.

1. Microeconomics (Price Theory)

Microeconomics studies the economic behaviour of **individual consumers**, **individual firms**, or **specific groups** (e.g., a group of dairy farmers or pet food producers). It focuses on how decisions are made at a smaller scale and how these decisions affect the allocation of resources.

Key Aspects of Microeconomics

1. **Individual Behaviour**: Examines the **economic behaviour of individual consumers, farms, or specific industries** (e.g., dairy, poultry, and pet food industry).
2. **Price Determination**: Examines how the prices of individual commodities (e.g., milk, eggs, pet food) or factors of production (e.g., labour, land) are determined. Example: How prices of chicken are set via supply or demand?
3. **Market Interactions**: Analyses demand and supply in specific markets –dairy/poultry.
4. **Theories**: covers **consumer behaviour theory** (what to buy), **price theory** (why eggs cost Rs 5), **and economic welfare theory** (are resources used well?).

2. Macroeconomics (Aggregative Economics)

Macroeconomics studies the **overall economy**, analysing broad factors such as national income, inflation, employment, and economic policies. It focuses on aggregate measures rather than individual units.

Key Aspects of Macroeconomics

i. **Big Scale**: Concerned with **large-scale economic activities** rather than individual firms or consumers.

ii. **Aggregates**: Examines **total income, total expenditure, total employment, and overall price levels (inflation),** the stuff of news stories & govt. policy debates.

iii. **Growth & Employment**: Studies **economic growth, income distribution, and employment levels** in a country.

iv. **Policy**: Helps in **policy formulation and economic analysis** to address issues like recession, inflation, and unemployment.

v. **Theories**: Theory of income &employment, theory of economic growth, policy formulation & analysis is studied.

Example

If a country experiences high inflation, the central bank may raise interest rates to reduce money supply and curb price rises. This could slow down economic growth but stabilize prices.

Key Differences between Microeconomics and Macroeconomics

Aspect	Microeconomics	Macroeconomics
Focus	Individual consumers, firms, or specific markets	Entire economy, aggregates
Scope	Small-scale economic activities	Large-scale economic phenomena
Key Variables	Prices, demand, supply of specific goods	GDP, inflation, unemployment, national income
Examples	Milk at Rs 50/L, egg demand	Economic growth, inflation rates, trade balance
Policy Implications	Affects individual markets and firms	Affects the overall economy and national policies

Economics: A Positive or Normative Science?

Economics isn't just one thing—it's a blend of **Positive Science** (what is), **Normative Science** (what ought to be), and **Applied Science** (how to get there). Each lens offers a different way to study wealth, resources, and human behaviour.

1. Economics as a Positive Science

A **positive science** explains economic phenomena as they are without making value judgments. It focuses on cause-and-effect relationships based on empirical data and objective analysis. A **positive science** is concerned with objective analysis and the study of "what is." It focuses on understanding and explaining economic phenomena based on facts, data, and empirical evidence, without making value judgments.

Characteristics of Positive Science

1. **Explains Why**: Digs into causes—like why egg prices spike. It explains the **"why" and "wherefore"** of economic issues. Why does inflation occur? What are the effects of unemployment?

2. **Describes Reality**: Describes the **current economic situation ("what is")** without suggesting solutions. India's GDP grew by 7% last year.
3. **Data-Driven**: Deals with **facts, data, and observations** to explain economic problems and their causes.
4. **Predictive**: It does not prescribe what should be done but, rather explains what is happening or what will happen if? Says what might happen if X changes—neutral analysis

Examples of Positive Economics

India's GDP grew by 7% last year in 2024 → this is an objective fact based on statistical data.

1. **A small percentage of people are very rich, while a large population remains poor** → this describes economic inequality without suggesting solutions.
2. **The price of milk rises when demand increases and supply is low** → this explains a market trend based on economic principles.

2. Economics as a Normative Science

A normative science is concerned with value judgments and «what ought to be.» It evaluates economic situations and prescribes solutions or policies solutions for economic problems.

Characteristics of Normative Science:

i. **Value Judgments**: Discusses the **rightness or wrongness** of economic issues. For example: Is income inequality fair? Should the government provide free healthcare or subsidised veterinary services?

ii. **Prescriptive**: Suggests **remedial measures** to solve economic problems. For example "The government should provide free vaccinations for all livestock to improve rural livelihoods.

iii. **Ideal Goals**: Defines **ideal economic conditions** to strive for. Reducing poverty, achieving full employment, or promoting sustainable agriculture.

iv. **Subjective and Value-Based**: Shaped by ethics, beliefs—not just facts.

   1. Example: "Antibiotic usage should be reduced in livestock farming to promote sustainable agriculture."

Examples of Normative Economics

1. The government should implement policies to reduce the rich-poor gap.
2. Free education and healthcare should be provided to all citizens.

3. Livestock farmers should adopt organic farming practices to protect the environment.

3. Economics as an Applied Science

Economics is also an **applied science** because it bridges the gap between **positive science** (what is) and **normative science** (what ought to be). It provides practical solutions and methods to achieve economic ideals.

Characteristics

- **Data to Policy:** Takes positive findings (e.g., inequality stats) and crafts normative solutions (e.g., subsidies).
- **Real-World Fixes:** Designs strategies to hit economic targets—jobs, sustainability.

Examples of Applied Economics

1. Designing policies to increase employment, such as promoting small-scale industries or providing vocational training.

Example of Positive, Normative and applied Economics

Milk Supply

- Positive: "Milk production fell 10% due to drought."
- Normative: "Farmers *ought* to get water aid."
- Applied: "Subsidize Rs 10,000 borewells—milk supply rebounds 8%."

Antibiotic Reduction

- Positive: "70% of poultry farms use antibiotics—resistance up 20%."
- Normative: "We *should* cut antibiotic use for sustainability."
- Applied: "Ban non-essential antibiotics, fund herbal alternatives—resistance drops 10% in 2 years."

Key Takeaways

- **Positive:** Facts—no judgment, just "milk is Rs 50/L because supply's tight."
- **Normative:** Values—"farmers should get fair prices."
- **Applied:** Action—"tax relief lifts small farms 10%."
- **Combo:** Economics explains (positive), dreams (normative), and does (applied)—vital for your farm

Characteristics of Economic Laws

Economic laws are fundamental principles that describe and predict economic behaviour and phenomena. Unlike laws in the natural sciences, economic laws are not exact or rigid. They are based on human behaviour, which is complex and variable. Below are the key characteristics of economic laws:

1. Economic Laws Are Not Exact

Economic laws are **generalizations** of human behaviour and are not certain or definite. This is because:

a) **Social, Legal, and Institutional Factors**: Human behaviour is influenced by social norms, legal frameworks, and institutional structures, which vary across societies and time.

b) **Variability of Human Actions**: Human actions are not always predictable, as they are influenced by emotions, preferences, and external factors.

c) **Lack of Controlled Experiments**: Unlike natural sciences, economics cannot conduct experiments under exact, controlled conditions. Economic phenomena are influenced by numerous variables that cannot be isolated.

Economic Laws Are Not Exact: Example

The law of demand states that, all else being equal, as the price of a good rises, the quantity demanded falls. However, this law may not hold true in all cases due to factors like changes in consumer preferences, income levels, or the availability of substitutes. Despite this, economics is more exact than other social sciences because economic phenomena can often be measured quantitatively (e.g., GDP, inflation rates, unemployment rates).

Example in Vet/Animal Husbandry

- **Law of Demand:** "Price up, demand down." Milk rises from Rs 50/L to Rs 60/L—demand drops from 100L to 80L, usually. But if a festival hits (shift factor), demand might stay at 100L—people splurge anyway.
- **Still Measurable:** Economics beats other social sciences with numbers—GDP, milk sales, vet fees—making it "more exact" than, say, sociology.

Key Insight

Your farm's milk sales might dip with a price hike—but a drought or fad could flip that. Expect trends, not guarantees.

2. Economic Laws Are Statements of Tendencies

Economic laws describe **tendencies** rather than absolute truths. They indicate how individuals or groups are likely to behave under certain conditions, but they do not guarantee that behavior will always follow the predicted pattern.

Example: The **law of supply** states that producers tend to supply more of a good when its price rises. However, this tendency may not hold if producers face constraints like resource shortages or production bottlenecks.

3. Economic Laws Are Qualified by the Assumption of *Ceteris Paribus*

Economic laws are **hypothetical** and hold true only under specific conditions. The assumption of *ceteris paribus* (Latin for "all other things being equal") is crucial in economics. It means that economic laws are valid only if all other factors remain constant.

Example: The law of demand states that demand for a good decrease as its price increases, *ceteris paribus*. However, if consumer income increases simultaneously, demand may not decrease despite the price rise.

4. Economic Laws Assume Rational Behaviour

Economic laws assume that individuals behave **rationally**. Rational behaviour means that individuals make decisions to maximize their satisfaction or utility, given their preferences and constraints.

Example: The **law of diminishing marginal utility** assumes that consumers allocate their income in a way that maximizes their total utility. However, human behaviour may not always be rational due to biases, emotions, or lack of information.

Example of a Vet Choice: Rational Pet Owner picks a Rs 500 vet over Rs 700—same care, lower cost. But loyalty to a pricier vet (emotion) breaks the rule.

5. Economic Laws Are Positive, Not Normative

Economic laws are **positive statements** that describe economic phenomena and establish cause-and-effect relationships. They do not make value judgments or prescribe what ought to be.

1. **Positive Statements**: These are factual and can be tested or verified using data. Example: "An increase in the minimum wage leads to higher unemployment."
2. **Normative Statements**: These involve value judgments and opinions about what should be done. Example: "The government should raise the minimum wage to reduce poverty."

Economic laws focus on **what is** rather than **what ought to be**.

Examples of Economic Laws

1. **Law of Demand**: As the price of a good increases, the quantity demanded decreases, *ceteris paribus*.
2. **Law of Supply**: As the price of a good increases, the quantity supplied increases, *ceteris paribus*.
3. **Law of Diminishing Marginal Utility**: As a consumer consumes more units of a good, the additional satisfaction (utility) derived from each additional unit decreases.
4. **Law of Diminishing Returns**: In production, adding more of one input while holding others constant will eventually yield smaller increases in output.

While economic laws are not as precise as laws in the natural sciences, they are essential for analyzing economic behavior, formulating policies, and making informed decisions. By understanding these characteristics, economists can better interpret economic phenomena and address real-world challenges.

Analytical Questions and Answers

Question 1

Define the traditional approach to the study of economics. What are its four components?

Answer

The traditional approach divides economics into four interconnected components: **Consumption**, **Production**, **Exchange**, and **Distribution** (CPED).

- **Consumption:** Use of goods/services (e.g., drinking milk, using vet services).
- **Production:** Creation of goods/services using land, labor, capital, and organization.
- **Exchange:** Buying/selling (e.g., farmer selling milk to a cooperative).
- **Distribution:** Allocation of income among landowners, laborers, capital providers, and entrepreneurs.

Question 2

What is consumption in economics? Give examples from animal husbandry.

Answer

Consumption refers to the use of goods and services to satisfy needs, leading to utility destruction (once used, it can't be reused).

Examples

- Drinking 5L of milk/week (Rs 50/L) or eating eggs—nutrients consumed, utility ends.
- Paying Rs 500 for a vet to vaccinate a cow—the service is consumed.

Question 3

Explain the concept of production and mention the four factors of production with dairy examples.

Answer

Production involves transforming resources into goods/services to create utility. The four factors are:

1. **Land:** E.g., 10 acres of grazing land.
2. **Labour:** E.g., Workers milking 20 cows.
3. **Capital:** E.g., Rs 50,000 for a milking machine.
4. **Organization:** E.g., Farmer managing feeding and milking for 500L/week output.

Question 4

What is the difference between microeconomics and macroeconomics?

Answer

Aspect	Microeconomics	Macroeconomics
Focus	Individual firms, consumers, markets	Entire economy and aggregates
Scope	Small-scale	Large-scale
Key Variables	Prices, supply, demand	GDP, inflation, employment
Examples	Milk at Rs 50/L, egg demand	National income growth, trade balance
Policy Implications	Affects specific sectors	Impacts national policy and economy

Question 5

Distinguish between positive, normative, and applied economics using examples

Answer

Type	Meaning	Example – Milk Supply
Positive	Describes 'what is' using facts	"Milk production fell 10% due to drought."
Normative	Describes 'what ought to be' based on values	"Farmers should get water aid."
Applied	Applies theory to real problems	"Subsidize borewells to increase supply."

Question 6

What is distribution in traditional economics? How is it seen in a dairy farm setup?

Answer

Distribution is the allocation of income among the four production factors. Dairy Farm Example

- **Landowner** earns rent.
- **Laborers** earn wages (e.g., for milking, feeding).
- **Capitalist** earns interest on machinery.
- **Entrepreneur (farmer)** earns profit by managing the operations.

Question 7

How does modern economics view the subject? Explain with an example from veterinary science.

Answer

Modern economics has two branches: **Microeconomics** and **Macroeconomics**.

- Micro: Studies individual vet clinics—pricing of ultrasound scans, demand for vaccinations.
- Macro: Looks at national policies on livestock subsidies, vet employment rates, or inflation in animal feed prices.

Question 8

Why is economics considered a science? What kind of science is it?

Answer

Economics is considered a science because it uses **data, theory, and analysis** to understand real-world economic problems.

- It is a **Positive Science**: Studies facts without judgment.
- A **Normative Science**: Suggests what *should* happen.
- An **Applied Science**: Provides practical solutions.

Question 9

Give an example each of a positive, normative, and applied economic statement in poultry farming.

Answer

- **Positive:** "70% of poultry farms use antibiotics."
- **Normative:** "We should reduce antibiotic usage in poultry."
- **Applied:** "Fund herbal alternatives and regulate non-essential antibiotic use."

Question 10

What role does exchange play in economic activity? Illustrate with examples.

Answer

Exchange involves the legal and ethical transfer of goods/services, facilitating the link between producers and consumers.

Examples

- Dairy farmer sells milk to cooperative or online platform.
- Vet pharmacy sells dewormers to farmers.
- Poultry farm sells eggs in local markets or exports them.

Question 11

How can the Traditional Approach's focus on Consumption help a dairy farmer decide whether to sell milk directly to consumers or to a cooperative?

Answer

The Traditional Approach's Consumption aspect studies how goods and services are used to satisfy needs, involving the destruction of utility. For a dairy farmer producing 500L of milk weekly (Rs 50/L), this means analyzing how consumers utilize milk—whether it is drunk directly (utility gone after consumption) or processed into products like cheese. Selling directly to consumers might fetch Rs 25,000/week (500L × Rs 50), but requires effort in marketing and delivery, and some milk might spoil if demand dips. Selling to a cooperative could offer a lower price (e.g., Rs 45/L = Rs 22,500/week) but ensures stable demand and less waste, as the co-op handles distribution. Consumption insights show the endgame is meeting human needs—direct sales maximize revenue if local demand is high, while co-ops align with bulk utility destruction. The farmer must weigh income against logistical ease, reflecting consumption's role in economic decisions.

Question 12

Using the Production component of the Traditional Approach, how might a poultry farmer optimize egg output with limited resources?

Answer

Production in the Traditional Approach involves transforming resources into goods/services using Land, Labour, Capital, and Organisation. For a poultry farmer with 1,000 hens on 1 acre (as per your example), optimization means coordinating these factors efficiently. Land (1 acre) limits flock size, so rotational grazing or multi-tier cages could maximize space. Labour (3 workers feeding hens) could be trained to monitor health, boosting egg yield from 700/day to 800/day (Rs 5/egg = Rs 4,000/day). Capital (Rs 20,000 feed stock) might shift to cheaper, nutrient-rich alternatives, cutting costs to Rs 15,000 while maintaining output. Organisation (the farmer) schedules feeding and collection to minimize waste—e.g., twice-daily checks. This creates more utility (eggs) from scarce resources, aligning with Production's goal. The trade-off is initial investment vs. long-term gains, requiring smart resource management.

Question 13

How does the Exchange process in the Traditional Approach explain the benefits of a veterinary pharmacy selling medicines online versus in-store?

Answer

Exchange involves transferring ownership of goods/services, historically via barter, now through money-based markets. For a veterinary pharmacy, selling medicines (e.g., Rs 500 vaccines) in-store limits reach to local farmers, say 20 sales/week (Rs 10,000). Online sales, as your chapter notes, tap into broader markets—potentially 50 sales/week (Rs 25,000) across regions or countries. Money as a medium scales this efficiently, unlike barter (e.g., trading vaccines for milk). Benefits include higher revenue, wider access for livestock owners, and inventory turnover, facilitating flow from producer (pharmacy) to consumer (farmers). However, online sales require capital (website, shipping) and organisation (logistics), per the Traditional Approach. In-store offers personal trust but caps growth. Exchange highlights how market choice impacts reach and profit in vet services.

Question 14

In the context of Distribution under the Traditional Approach, how should a dairy farm owner allocate profits among factors of production during a bumper milk year?

Answer

Distribution shares production earnings among Land, Labour, Capital, and Organisation based on contribution (factor pricing). In a bumper year, a dairy farm with 20 cows produces 600L/week (vs. 500L normally) at Rs 50/L, earning Rs 30,000/week. The landowner might get Rs 5,000 rent (grazing land value rises with output). Workers (2 milkers) could earn Rs 8,000 wages (extra effort for higher yield). Capital (investor's Rs 50,000 milking machine) might claim Rs 3,000 interest, reflecting its role in efficiency. The owner (Organisation) takes Rs 14,000 profit for managing sales and risks—higher than usual due to the surplus. This allocation rewards each factor's input, per your vet clinic example (rent, interest, wages, profit). The owner must balance reinvestment (e.g., new equipment) with fair payouts, ensuring future productivity.

Question 15

How can Microeconomics help a veterinarian set competitive prices for pet ultrasound services in a small town?

Answer

Microeconomics, as your Modern Approach explains, studies individual behavior and price determination via supply and demand. For a vet offering ultrasound services (Rs 10,000 tool, 20 visits/week at Rs 500 each = Rs 10,000 revenue), setting a competitive price means analyzing local pet owners (consumers) and rival vets (supply). If demand is high (50 pet owners/week) but only two vets offer ultrasounds, scarcity drives prices up—say, Rs 600 (Rs 12,000/week). If a third vet enters, supply rises, potentially dropping prices to Rs 450 to retain clients (Rs 9,000/week). Microeconomics' price theory helps the vet test: "What price balances costs (Rs 2,000/week for tool loan, rent) with demand?" A Rs 500 sweet spot maximizes welfare (pet health) and profit, showing how individual market interactions guide pricing.

Question 16

Using Macroeconomics, how might a national recession impact a dairy farmer's decision to expand herd size?

Answer

Macroeconomics studies aggregates like GDP, employment, and inflation, per your chapter. In a recession, national income falls, unemployment rises, and consumers cut spending—e.g., milk demand drops from 500L/week to 400L at Rs 50/L (Rs 20,000 vs. Rs 25,000). Feed costs might rise due to inflation (Rs 10/kg to Rs 12/kg), squeezing margins. Expanding the herd (e.g., 20 to 25 cows) requires capital (Rs 50,000/cow = Rs 250,000), but lower demand and higher costs risk losses. Macro policy—like your interest rate example—might tighten loans, making expansion costlier. The farmer might delay, focusing on efficiency (e.g., better fodder use) until GDP recovers, showing how big-scale trends shape farm decisions.

Question 17

How does Positive Economics differ from Normative Economics when analyzing a drop in milk production due to drought, and what might Applied Economics suggest?

Answer

Positive Economics describes "what is" with facts, per your chapter. For a drought cutting milk from 500L to 450L/week (10% drop), it states: "Drought reduced water, lowering cow yield." Normative Economics adds value judgments—"Farmers ought to get subsidies to offset losses"—prescribing ideals. Positive is data-driven (e.g., yield stats), while Normative is subjective (fairness debate). Applied Economics bridges them: using the 10% drop fact, it might propose, "Subsidize Rs 10,000 borewells—milk rebounds 8% (480L/week)." Your milk supply example fits perfectly—Positive explains, Normative dreams, Applied acts. This helps vets/farmers understand causes, set goals, and find solutions.

Question 18

How can a vet use Applied Economics to address antibiotic overuse in poultry, considering Positive and Normative insights?

Answer

Positive Economics notes: "70% of poultry farms use antibiotics—resistance up 20%" (your example)—a fact. Normative Economics counters: "We should cut antibiotic use for sustainability"—a goal. Applied Economics acts: "Ban non-essential antibiotics, fund herbal alternatives—resistance drops 10% in 2 years." A vet could implement this by advising farmers to switch to probiotics (Rs 5,000 initial cost vs. Rs 3,000 antibiotics), using Positive data (resistance trends) to justify the Normative ideal (healthier flocks). Revenue might dip short-term (fewer quick fixes), but long-term gains (market trust, lower resistance) align with your chapter's real-world fix focus. This blends analysis, values, and action for poultry health.

3

Basic Terms and Concepts in Economics

Economics revolves around key concepts such as goods **value**, **price**, **wealth**, **income**, **savings**, **investment**, and **consumption**.

These concepts are interconnected and form the foundation of economic analysis. Below is a detailed explanation of each:

Goods: Definition, Types, and Economic Importance

Definition of Goods

Goods refer to **tangible or intangible items** that satisfy human wants and have value. Goods can be material (physical objects) or non-material (services), and they play a crucial role in fulfilling human needs and desires. They form the basis of **economic activity**, as humans constantly seek to fulfil their needs and desires.

Examples

Tangible Goods: You can touch them. Food, clothing, vehicles, dairy products.

Intangible Goods (Services): Services you experience. Veterinary services, teaching, medical care.

Classification of Goods in Economics

Goods can be categorized based on different criteria such as material nature, supply, transferability, consumption, ownership, and income elasticity.

1. According to Material or Non-Material Nature

a) Material Goods

i. These are **tangible** and physical items that can be seen, touched, and stored.

ii. They are the concrete outcomes of production and have the power to satisfy human wants.

iii. **Examples**: Land, buildings, furniture, clothes, food, electronics.

b) Non-Material Goods

i. These are **intangible** and cannot be touched or stored. They are often services provided by individuals or institutions.

ii. **Examples**

- Services of a doctor (healthcare).
- Services of a teacher (education).
- Services of a veterinarian (animal healthcare).
- Banking services, AI services, training programs

2. According to Their Supply

a) Free Goods

i. These are goods that exist in **abundance** and are available without cost.

ii. They do not require human effort or sacrifice to produce.

iii. **Examples**: Air, sunlight, seawater.

iv. **Note**: The distinction between free goods and economic goods can blur over time. For example, clean drinking water, once a free good, has become an economic good in many regions due to scarcity.

b) Economic Goods

i. These are **scarce** goods that require human effort, resources, and sacrifice to produce.

ii. They have an **opportunity cost** (the cost of the next best alternative foregone) and command a price in the market.

iii. **Examples**: Cars, smartphones, clothes, machinery.

iv. **Characteristics**:

a) Produced through human effort.

b) Limited in quantity.

c) Have a price and are traded in markets.

3. According to Transferability

a) Transferable Goods

i. These are goods whose **ownership can be transferred** from one person to another.

ii. Most **material goods** fall under this category.

iii. **Examples**: Cars, houses, books, electronics.

b) Non-Transferable Goods

i. These are goods whose **ownership cannot be physically transferred**.

ii. They often include **intangible goods** like skills, abilities, or intelligence.

iii. **Examples**

a) Skills (e.g., a doctor's expertise).

b) A vet's diagnostic skill.

c) Intelligence or talent (e.g., a musician's ability).

d) Personal traits (e.g., charisma).

4. According to Consumption

a) Consumer Goods

i. These are goods that are **directly used by consumers** to satisfy their wants.

ii. They provide immediate satisfaction and are not used for further production.

iii. **Types of Consumer Goods**:

a) Durable Goods: Goods that last for a long time and can be used repeatedly (e.g., furniture, cars, electronics, fridge for milk storage, boots for farm work

b) Non-Durable Goods: Goods that are consumed quickly (e.g., food, milk, eggs).

iv. **Examples**: Clothes, shoes, bread, meat, milk.

b) Capital Goods (Producer Goods)

i. These are goods used to **produce other goods and services**. They do not directly satisfy consumer wants but are essential for production.

ii. **Examples**: Machinery, tools, raw materials, livestock (used for dairy or meat production) Milking machines, plows, breeding bulls, vet tools.

c) Public and Private Goods

i. **Public Goods**: Owned by the government or society and available to all (e.g., streetlights, national defence).

ii. **Private Goods**: Owned by individuals or private entities (e.g., personal cars, houses).

d) Complementary and Substitute Goods

i. **Complementary Goods**: Goods that are used together (e.g., tea and sugar, cars and fuel, Rural roads, animal disease control programs.).

ii. **Substitute Goods**: Goods that can replace each other (e.g., tea and coffee, soybean meal and fish meal in animal feed).

Based on Income Elasticity

a) Normal Goods

i. Demand for these goods **increases as income rises**.

ii. **Examples**: Luxury cars, branded clothes, high-quality food.

b) Inferior Goods

i. Demand for these goods **decreases as income rises**.

ii. **Examples**: Low-quality rice, second-hand goods, low-cost animal feed.

c) Luxury Goods

i. Demand for these goods **increases more than proportionally as income rises**.

ii. **Examples**: Designer clothes, high-end electronics, luxury vacations.

Conclusion

Goods can be categorized based on their **material nature**, **supply**, **transferability**, and **consumption patterns**. Understanding these categories helps in analysing economic behaviour, production processes, and market dynamics. Key takeaways include:

1. **Material vs. Non-Material Goods**: Tangible vs. intangible.
2. **Free vs. Economic Goods**: Abundance vs. scarcity.
3. **Transferable vs. Non-Transferable Goods**: Ownership transferability.
4. **Consumer vs. Capital Goods**: Direct vs. indirect satisfaction of wants.
5. **Utility**: The ability of a good to satisfy human wants.
6. **Income Elasticity**: How demand for goods changes with income (normal, inferior, luxury goods).

Conclusion: Why This Matters

Understanding goods helps you analyse

i. **Material vs. Non-Material:** Feed vs. vet advice—both keep farms running.
ii. **Free vs. Economic:** Air's free, but milk costs effort—scarcity drives value.
iii. **Transferable vs. Non-Transferable:** Sell a cow, not your skill.
iv. **Consumer vs. Capital:** Eggs feed people; machines make eggs possible.
v. **Utility:** Goods satisfy wants—core of economics.
vi. **Income Elasticity:** Richer farmers demand better—know your market.

1. Goods are tangible (cows) or intangible (vet skills).
2. They're free (sunlight) or economic (feed), transferable (eggs) or not (talent).
3. Consumption splits them into consumer (milk) or capital (tractors).
4. Income tweaks demand—normal, inferior, or luxury.

2. Utility: The Want-Satisfying Power of a Good

Utility refers to the ability of a good or service to satisfy a human want. It is a subjective concept and varies from person to person and asks one simple question: *"Does it meet a need or desire?"* If yes, it's got utility; if not, it doesn't.

Utility and Usefulness

In economics, **utility** refers to the ability of a good or service to satisfy a human want or need. It is important to note that utility is not the same as **usefulness**. A good may have utility even if it is not useful or even harmful. For example, intoxicating liquor or cigarettes may satisfy a human want, and people are willing to pay for them, so they possess utility in economic terms, even though their consumption may be injurious to health. Thus, the concept of utility in economics is **neutral** and has no ethical or moral significance.

Characteristics of Utility

1. **Utility is Subjective**: Utility varies from person to person based on their preferences, needs, and circumstances.

   Example

   i. A smoker derives utility from cigarettes, while a non-smoker does not.

   ii. A dairy farmer may find Artificial Insemination (AI) services highly useful, while a poultry farmer may have no interest in them.

2. **Utility is Not Synonymous with Pleasure**: A good or service may have utility even if it does not provide pleasure.

   Example

   i. Bitter medicines are difficult to swallow and may not provide pleasure, but they fulfil a need and thus have utility.

ii. Vaccination may be painful for animals and inconvenient for farmers, but it has utility as it prevents diseases.

3. **Utility Does Not Always Mean Satisfaction**: A person may not be fully satisfied after consuming a product, but the product still holds utility as it fulfills a need.

   Example

   i. A dairy farmer may vaccinate his animals as a preventive measure, but he may still be unsatisfied if the milk yield does not improve. The vaccine has utility because it prevents disease, even if the farmer is not fully satisfied.

4. **Utility Varies with Time, Place, and Situation**

   The utility of a good or service can change depending on the time, place, and situation.

   Examples

   i. An umbrella has more utility during the rainy season than in summer.

   ii. Water has different utilities when used for drinking, bathing, or washing.

   iii. Veterinary medicines have higher utility during disease outbreaks but lower utility in disease-free periods.

Types of Utility

Utility can be created or enhanced in various ways. The four main types of utility are:

1. **Form Utility**: Created by changing the form or shape of a good to make it more useful.

   Example

   i. Milk to Cheese: Turning liquid milk into milk powder or cheese.

   ii. Wool to Blanket**:** Raw wool (Rs 100/kg) turns into a Rs 500 blanket—utility jumps.

2. **Place Utility**: Created by transporting goods to places where they are needed or valued more.

   Example

   Rural to Urban Milk: 100L milk from a village (Rs 40/L) hits city shelves (Rs 60/L)—place utility cashes in.

   i. Exporting veterinary medicines to regions experiencing disease outbreaks.

3. **Time Utility**: Created by making goods available when they are needed. This often involves storage.

   Example

   i. Storing fodder for livestock during the dry season.

   ii. Stockpiling vaccines for future disease outbreaks.

4. **Possession Utility**: Created by transferring ownership of goods to those who value them the most.

   Example

   i. Selling livestock to farmers who need them for dairy or meat production.

   ii. Transferring ownership of veterinary equipment to clinics.

Key Differences between Utility and Usefulness

Aspect	**Utility**	**Usefulness**
Definition	Ability of a good or service to satisfy a human want or need.	Practical value or benefit of a good or service.
Ethical/Moral Aspect	Neutral – No ethical or moral significance.	Often associated with positive or beneficial outcomes.
Examples	Cigarettes have utility for smokers but are not useful for health.	Medicines are useful for treating diseases and improving health.
Subjectivity	Varies from person to person based on preferences and needs.	Generally objective and based on practical benefits.

Conclusion

i. **Utility** in economics refers to the ability of a good or service to satisfy a human want or need, regardless of whether it is useful or harmful.

ii. It is a **subjective** concept that varies from person to person and depends on time, place, and situation.

iii. Utility is not the same as **pleasure** or **satisfaction**, and it does not always imply usefulness.

iv. Utility can be created or enhanced through **form**, **place**, **time**, and **possession**.

Understanding the concept of utility helps in analyzing consumer behavior, production decisions, and market dynamics. It provides insights into why people choose certain goods and services over others, even when those choices may not align with traditional notions of usefulness or morality.

Utility: Snippet

Utility is the ability of a good or service to satisfy a human want—it's the "want-satisfying juice" in anything we consume. It's subjective, varying person to person.

Utility isn't about being "good" or "useful"—it's neutral. A cigarette satisfies a smoker's craving (utility), even if it trashes their lungs (not useful). Economics doesn't judge—it just measures the want fulfilled.

3. Value

Value refers to the worth of a good or service and in economics can be understood in two main ways:

a) Value in Use

i. This refers to the **utility** or satisfaction derived from consuming a good or service.

ii. **Example**: Fresh air and sunshine have great value in use because they provide utility, even though they are free.

b) Value in Exchange

i. This refers to the **ability of a good or service to be exchanged for other goods or services**.

ii. It is the **purchasing power** of a commodity in terms of other commodities.

iii. **Example**: A liter of milk can be exchanged for a loaf of bread.

iv. **Note**

Free goods (e.g., air, sunlight) have **value in use** but no **value in exchange**.

Economic goods (e.g., milk, clothes) have both **value in use** and **value in exchange**.

Attributes of Value

For a good to have value, it must satisfy three conditions:

i. **Utility**: It must satisfy a human want or need.

ii. **Scarcity**: It must be limited in supply.

iii. **Transferability**: It must be marketable or transferable.

4. Price

i. Price is the **monetary amount** at which a good or service is exchanged in the market.

ii. It is the **value of a good expressed in terms of money**.

iii. **Factors Influencing Price**:
   1. Supply and demand.
   2. Market conditions (e.g., competition, monopolies).
   3. Government intervention (e.g., subsidies, taxes).

iv. **Example**: If the price of milk is ₹50 per liter, it means milk can be exchanged for ₹50 in the market.

5. Wealth

i. In economics, **wealth** refers to the total stock of **valuable assets** owned by an individual, firm, or nation.

ii. It includes:
   a) **Physical assets**: Land, buildings, machinery, livestock.
   b) **Financial assets**: Cash, stocks, bonds.
   c) **Intangible assets**: Intellectual property, skills, knowledge.

Classification of Wealth

1. **Individual Wealth**
   i. Material goods (e.g., cash, land, livestock).
   ii. Non-material goods (e.g., goodwill, patents).
2. **Personal Wealth**

   Personal qualities like skills, abilities, and intelligence are not wealth because they are not salable.
3. **Social or Communal Wealth**

   Assets owned by society (e.g., roads, public parks, hospitals).
4. **National Wealth**

   The aggregate wealth of a nation, excluding debts owed to one another.

   Includes natural resources (e.g., rivers, mountains).
5. **Cosmopolitan Wealth**

   The total wealth of all nations combined.
6. **Negative Wealth**

   Debts owed by individuals or states.

6. Income

i. Income is the **flow of value** generated by wealth over a period.

ii. It is what wealth yields and is distributed among the factors of production (land, labor, capital, and entrepreneurship) in the form of:

a) **Rent** (for land).

b) **Wages** (for labor).

c) **Interest** (for capital).

d) **Profit** (for entrepreneurship).

Types of Income

i. Money Income: Income measured in monetary terms (e.g., a farmer earns ₹5,000 from selling milk).

ii. Real Income

a) The **purchasing power** of money income, adjusted for inflation.

b) Reflects the actual goods and services a person can buy.

iii. Generated Income: Income earned by contributing to the production process (e.g., wages, rent, interest, profit).

iv. Transfer Income: Income received without contributing to production (e.g., pensions, scholarships).

v. National Income: The total income generated by a nation's economic activities.

7. Savings

i. Savings refer to the **excess of income over consumption**.

ii. It can be held in the form of cash, bank balances, or investments.

iii. Formula

Savings = Income − Consumption

8. Investment

i. Investment refers to the **addition made to a nation's physical capital**.

ii. It includes:

1. Building new factories.
2. Purchasing new machinery.
3. Adding to the stock of finished goods.

iii. Formula

Income = Consumption + Investment

9. Consumption

i. Consumption refers to the **satisfaction of wants** by using goods and services.

ii. It involves the **destruction of utility** (e.g., eating food, wearing clothes).

Types of Consumption

i. Direct or Final Consumption: Goods are used to satisfy human wants directly (e.g., eating a mango, wearing a shirt).

ii. Indirect Consumption: Goods are used to produce other goods (e.g., using a sewing machine to make clothes).

iii. Useful vs. Wasteful Consumption

Useful Consumption: Goods are used to satisfy wants (e.g., drinking water to quench thirst).

Wasteful Consumption: Goods are destroyed without satisfying wants (e.g., destruction by fire or natural calamities).

Conclusion

i. Value is the worth of a good or service, measured in terms of utility (value in use) or exchange (value in exchange).

ii. Price is the monetary expression of value.

iii. Wealth is the stock of valuable assets, while **income** is the flow of value generated by wealth.

iv. Savings represent the portion of income not consumed, and **investment** refers to additions to physical capital.

v. Consumption is the act of using goods and services to satisfy wants.

These concepts are interconnected and form the basis of economic analysis, helping us understand how resources are allocated, utilized, and distributed in an economy.

10. Wants in Economics

In economics, **wants** refer to the desires for goods and services that are backed by the **ability and willingness to pay** for them. Wants are the driving force behind all economic activities, as they give rise to production, consumption, and exchange. Below is a detailed explanation of the concept of wants, their characteristics, and their classification.

1. Definition of Wants

i. Ordinary Sense: In everyday language, "wants" are often used interchangeably with "desires."

ii. **Economic Sense**: In economics, there is a fine distinction between the two:

   1. **Desire**: A conscious longing for something (e.g., a beggar desiring a car).
   2. **Want**: A desire that is backed by **purchasing power** (ability to pay) and **willingness to pay**.

   Example: A rich person desires a car, has the money to buy it, and is willing to pay for it. This is a **want**.

2. Attributes of Wants

For a desire to become a **want**, it must satisfy three conditions:

i. **Desire for a Good**: A conscious longing for a specific good or service.
ii. **Purchasing Power**: The ability to pay for the good or service.
iii. **Willingness to Pay**: The readiness to spend money to satisfy the desire.

When a desire is backed by purchasing power and willingness to pay, it becomes an **effective desire** or **want**. Effective desires form the basis of **demand** in economics.

3. Importance of Wants in Economics

i. Wants are the **seeds** that give rise to economic activities.
ii. The feeling of unmet wants leads to production, consumption, and exchange.
iii. As one want is satisfied, new wants emerge, ensuring that economic activities continue to grow.

4. Characteristics of Wants

i. **Wants are Unlimited**
   1. Human wants are endless. As one want is satisfied, another arises.
   2. **Example**: A person who has never owned a car desires one. Once they own a car, they may desire a bigger or more luxurious model.

ii. **Particular Wants Can Be Satisfied**:
   1. A specific want can be fully satisfied if the means are available.
   2. **Example**: A hungry person can satisfy their want for food by eating. A livestock farmer can satisfy the want for treating mastitis by providing medical care to the cow.

iii. Wants are Complementary

1. Often, one good alone cannot satisfy a want; complementary goods are needed.
2. **Example**: To write, you need both a pen and paper.

iv. Wants are Competitive

1. Since resources are limited, individuals must choose which wants to satisfy first.
2. **Example**: A farmer may prioritize buying fodder for animals over purchasing a new tractor.

v. Wants Vary in Urgency and Intensity

1. Some wants are more urgent and intense than others.
2. **Example**: A farmer facing a disease outbreak in livestock will prioritize treatment over long-term investments like a bulk milk cooler.

vi. Wants Have Alternative Means of Satisfaction:

1. There are often multiple ways to satisfy a want.
2. **Example**: Protein can be obtained from pulses, milk, eggs, or meat.

vii. Wants are Recurring

1. Many wants recur over time and require repeated satisfaction.
2. **Example**: A livestock farmer needs to feed animals regularly.

viii. Wants Vary with Time, Place, and Person

1. Wants differ based on individual preferences, location, and time.
2. **Example**: In hilly regions, livestock farmers may want heated shelters, while in plains, they may need cooling systems.

ix. Present Wants are More Important than Future Wants

1. People prioritize satisfying present wants over future wants.
2. **Example**: A dairy farmer facing a mastitis outbreak will focus on immediate treatment rather than long-term preventive measures.

x. Wants are Influenced by Income, Salesmanship, and Advertisement

1. Higher income increases the ability to satisfy wants.
2. Advertising and marketing influence the desire for goods and services.

5. Classification of Wants

Wants can be classified into three categories based on their importance and urgency:

1. **Necessaries**
    1. Wants that must be satisfied for survival or efficiency.
    2. **Types of Necessaries**
        i. **Necessaries of Existence**: Basic needs like food, clothing, and shelter.
        ii. **Necessaries of Efficiency**: Goods that improve productivity (e.g., a table and chair for students).
        iii. **Conventional Necessaries**: Goods required due to social customs (e.g., formal clothing for work).
2. **Comforts**
    i. Wants that provide a higher standard of living but are not essential for survival.
    ii. **Example**: Air conditioning, comfortable furniture.
3. **Luxuries**
    i. Wants that provide pleasure or status but are not necessary for survival or comfort.
    ii. **Example**: Designer clothes, luxury cars.

6. Economic Wants vs. Non-Economic Wants

1. **Economic Wants**
    i. Wants that can be satisfied by purchasing goods and services from the market.
    ii. **Example**: Buying food, clothing, or veterinary services.
2. **Non-Economic Wants**
    i. Wants that cannot be satisfied through market transactions.
    ii. **Example**: The desire for fresh air or love.

Conclusion

1. **Wants** are the foundation of all economic activities. They are desires backed by purchasing power and willingness to pay.
2. Wants are **unlimited**, **recurring**, and **vary in urgency and intensity**.
3. They can be classified into **necessaries**, **comforts**, and **luxuries** based on their importance.
4. Understanding wants helps in analyzing consumer behavior, production decisions, and market dynamics.

By studying wants, economists and businesses can better understand how to allocate resources, design products, and create policies that satisfy human needs and desires.

Short Questions

1. What are goods in economics?

Answer

Goods are tangible or intangible items that satisfy human wants and have value. They may be material (e.g., milk, tractors) or non-material (e.g., veterinary services, teaching).

2. Differentiate between material and non-material goods with examples.

Answer

- **Material Goods:** Tangible items like clothes, food, vehicles.
- **Non-Material Goods:** Intangible services like teaching, medical care, veterinary aid.

3. What is the difference between free goods and economic goods?

Answer

- **Free Goods:** Available in abundance without cost (e.g., sunlight, air).
- **Economic Goods:** Scarce, require resources to produce, and have a price (e.g., milk, clothes).

4. Explain transferable and non-transferable goods with examples.

Answer

- **Transferable Goods:** Ownership can be passed (e.g., cars, land).
- **Non-Transferable Goods:** Ownership cannot be passed (e.g., skills, intelligence).

5. Define consumer goods and capital goods with two examples each.

Answer

- **Consumer Goods:** Used directly for consumption (e.g., milk, eggs).
- **Capital Goods:** Used for further production (e.g., tractors, milking machines).

6. What are complementary and substitute goods? Give examples.

Answer

- **Complementary Goods:** Used together (e.g., tea and sugar, cars and fuel).
- **Substitute Goods:** Can replace each other (e.g., tea and coffee, fish meal and soybean meal in feed).

7. Explain normal, inferior, and luxury goods with examples.

Answer

- **Normal Goods:** Demand increases with income (e.g., milk, branded clothes).
- **Inferior Goods:** Demand decreases with income (e.g., low-cost feed, second-hand clothes).
- **Luxury Goods:** Demand rises more than proportionally with income (e.g., designer clothes, luxury cars).

8. Why is understanding the classification of goods important in economics?

Answer

It helps analyze economic behavior, guide production decisions, market demand, and tailor goods for different income levels and needs.

Section 2: Utility

9. What is utility in economics?

Answer

Utility is the ability of a good or service to satisfy a human want, regardless of its usefulness or ethical value.

10. Is utility the same as usefulness? Justify with examples.

Answer

No. Utility is about satisfying a want. Cigarettes may have utility for smokers but are not useful health-wise. Medicines are useful and also have utility.

11. What does it mean that utility is subjective?

Answer

Utility varies from person to person. A vet's AI service may be valuable to a dairy farmer but meaningless to a poultry farmer.

12. List and explain the four types of utility with examples.

Answer

1. **Form Utility:** Created by changing the shape/form (e.g., milk to cheese).
2. **Place Utility:** Created by transporting goods (e.g., milk from village to city).
3. **Time Utility:** Created by storing goods for later (e.g., fodder for dry season).
4. **Possession Utility:** Created by transferring ownership (e.g., selling animals).

13. Can a good have utility but not give satisfaction? Explain.

Answer

Yes. Vaccines may not give satisfaction (painful or no visible result), but they fulfill a need, hence have utility.

14. How does utility vary with time and place? Give two examples.

Answer

- Umbrellas are more useful during rains (time utility).
- Veterinary medicine is more useful during outbreaks (place/time utility).

Analytical Questions

1. Free vs. Economic Goods: Transitioning Clean Water into a Business Opportunity

Question

How can you develop a business model that transforms clean water into an affordable economic good for poultry and dairy farmers? Consider the opportunity cost of production and how you'd convince farmers to invest in your solution over traditional (now scarce) sources.

Answer

To turn clean water from a free good into an economic good, create a scalable purification and distribution business that balances affordability with profitability.

- **Business Model:** Install low-cost, solar-powered water purifiers at strategic community points (e.g., near poultry or dairy farms). Charge a subscription fee (e.g., ₹100/month per farmer) for unlimited access to purified water, keeping it cheaper than bottled alternatives (₹5/liter).

- **Opportunity Cost:** The cost of setting up purifiers (₹50,000/unit) and maintenance (₹5,000/year) is offset by not relying on expensive tanker deliveries or imported filters. Farmers' alternative—digging wells or buying bottled water—costs more in time and money.
- **Convincing Farmers:** Educate them with data: "Clean water cuts livestock disease by 20%, boosting milk/egg output by 15%." Offer a free 1-month trial to demonstrate healthier animals and higher yields.
- **Outcome:** Subscription model ensures steady revenue (e.g., 50 farmers x ₹100 = ₹5,000/month per unit), while farmers see water as an investment, not a cost. Scale by partnering with local co-operatives

2. Free Goods vs. Economic Goods in Poultry Farming

Question

How would you convince the farmer to invest in solar lighting? Use the concepts of free goods vs. economic goods and opportunity cost to justify the decision.

To convince the farmer to invest in solar lighting

Free Goods Limitations: Highlight that while sunlight is free, its inconsistency (e.g., winter shortages) leads to lost production (opportunity cost).

Economic Goods ROI: Cost-Benefit: ₹15,000 investment → 20% higher egg production → extra ₹30,000/year (assuming 500 birds produce 10,000 eggs/year at ₹ 3/egg).

Payback Period: 6 months.

Behavioral Nudge: Offer a free trial (install lights in one cooperative to show results) or EMI options to reduce upfront cost.

Key Takeaway: Convert free-good dependency into economic-good investment by quantifying lost income vs. gains.

3. Consumer vs. Capital Goods: Scaling a Dairy Equipment Venture

Question

How can you use the distinction between consumer and capital goods to educate farmers on long-term benefits (e.g., higher milk yield and quality) and boost sales? Propose a pricing or bundling strategy to make your capital goods more appealing ?

Answer

Position milking machines (capital goods) as profit drivers and milk storage containers (durable consumer goods) as quality enhancers to shift farmer perception.

- **Education Strategy:** Host demonstrations showing: "Milking machines save 2 hours/day and increase yield by 10% vs. hand-milking; containers preserve milk freshness, fetching ₹5/litre more." Highlight durability: "Machines last 5+ years vs. cans needing yearly replacement."
- **Pricing/Bundling:** Offer a "Dairy Starter Kit": milking machine (₹20,000) + container (₹5,000) at ₹23,000 (10% discount). Add a 0% interest EMI plan (₹1,916/month for 12 months) to lower the upfront cost barrier.
- **Outcome:** Farmers see capital goods as tools for growth, not expenses. Sales rise as EMI and bundling make premium products accessible, with demos proving Rate of Investment ROI (e.g., ₹5,000 extra monthly income).

4. Complementary and Substitute Goods: Innovating Poultry Feed Sales

Question

How can you leverage the concept of complementary goods (e.g., partnering with logistics providers) and counter the substitution effect to retain customers? Suggest a strategy to differentiate your feed from substitutes like soybean meal?

Answer

Strengthen your feed's value by pairing it with complementary goods and outshining substitutes through quality and convenience.

- **Complementary Goods Strategy:** Partner with rural logistics firms to offer free delivery for orders over 100kg. Pitch: "Reliable roads + our feed = healthier birds, faster." Bundle feed with free vet checkups (complementary service) to lock in loyalty.
- **Countering Substitution:** Differentiate with a unique selling point: "Our feed has 20% more digestible protein than soybean meal, proven to cut grow-out time by 5 days." Back it with farmer testimonials and a money-back guarantee.
- **Pricing Tweak:** Introduce a mid-tier feed at ₹45/kg (vs. ₹50/kg premium) to compete directly with soybean meal (₹40/kg), retaining price-sensitive customers.
- **Outcome:** Delivery and vet perks make your feed indispensable; quality focus pulls farmers back from substitutes. Sales stabilize, with 30% shifting to mid-tier.

5. Transferable vs. Non-Transferable Goods: Building a Veterinary Service Brand

Question

How can you combine your non-transferable skills (e.g., diagnostic expertise) with transferable goods (e.g., tools) to create a unique value proposition? Design a service package that highlights your skills' worth and justifies your tool pricing.

Answer

Merge your expertise with tools to offer a premium, all-in-one solution that competitors can't replicate.

- **Value Proposition:** "Get my diagnostic skills + the tools I trust for healthier livestock." Position your non-transferable expertise (e.g., spotting diseases early) as the key to maximizing tool effectiveness.
- **Service Package:** Launch a "Vet Care Bundle": ₹2,000/month includes 1 farm visit (diagnosis + treatment plan) + branded tools (e.g., ₹500 thermometer, ₹1,000 syringe kit) at a 20% discount. Tools alone cost ₹1,800, so the bundle saves money and ties farmers to your service.
- **Justification:** Show ROI: "Early diagnosis prevents 10% flock loss (₹5,000 value); my tools ensure accurate follow-through." Contrast with DIY risks: "Cheap tools miss subtle signs."
- **Outcome:** Farmers pay for your skill, not just tools, boosting retention (75% renewals) and justifying higher tool prices through bundled value.

6. Income Elasticity of Demand for Dairy Products

A dairy entrepreneur in his region sells two types of milk: standard milk (₹ 50/litre) and organic, grass-fed milk (₹ 75/litre). Recently, as the income levels of consumers increased, more people started purchasing organic milk, while demand for standard milk slightly declined.

Question

How does this shift reflect the concept of normal and luxury goods? What marketing strategies can the entrepreneur use to further capitalize on this trend?

Answer

The increased demand for **organic, grass-fed milk** shows that it is a **luxury good**, while standard milk is a **normal good**. As income rises, people prefer higher-quality products. The dairy entrepreneur can:

1. **Branding & Storytelling** – Emphasize health benefits, ethical sourcing, and farm-to-table freshness to reinforce the premium nature of organic milk.
2. **Subscription Models** – Offer weekly or monthly home delivery to lock in repeat customers.
3. **Expand Product Line** – Introduce organic ghee, paneer, and curd to capture a broader premium market.

This case highlights the **income elasticity of demand**—luxury goods see higher demand as income rises.

7. Subjective Utility: Tailoring Veterinary Services for Diverse Farmers

Question

You're a veterinarian offering disease prevention services (e.g., vaccinations) in a mixed farming region. Dairy farmers value your services highly for milk yield protection, but poultry farmers see little utility, preferring cheaper home remedies. How can you adjust your approach to increase the subjective utility of your services for poultry farmers without lowering prices?

Answer

Recognize that utility is subjective and varies by farmer type—dairy farmers see prevention as a yield-saver, while poultry farmers prioritize cost over long-term health.

i. **Strategy:** Shift poultry farmers' perception by targeting their specific wants: faster bird growth and higher egg output. Offer a "Poultry Health Package" with vaccinations plus a free growth-boosting supplement trial (e.g., vitamins worth ₹200).

ii. **Utility Boost:** Highlight data: "Vaccinated flocks grow 10% faster, adding ₹500 profit per cycle." This ties your service to their desire for quick returns, not just disease prevention.

iii. **Execution:** Host on-farm demos showing healthier birds post-vaccination, leveraging time utility (immediate results matter to them). Avoid price cuts—focus on perceived value.

iv. **Outcome:** Poultry farmers adopt your service (e.g., 20% uptake in 3 months), as subjective utility rises without compromising your margins.

8. Utility vs. Usefulness: Marketing a Controversial Poultry Product

Question

You're a poultry entrepreneur selling a high-energy feed additive that boosts egg production but has mild side effects (e.g., temporary feather loss). Farmers hesitate, arguing it's not "useful" due to health concerns, though some still buy it for profit gains. How can you market this additive by emphasizing its utility over its usefulness?

Answer

Utility is neutral—your additive satisfies the want for higher profits, even if it's not "useful" for bird health.

- **Strategy:** Pitch it as a profit tool, not a health product: "Boost egg output by 15% in 30 days—₹1,000 extra per flock." Acknowledge side effects transparently: "Feather loss is temporary; profits aren't."
- **Utility Focus:** Use possession utility—sell small batches (e.g., 5kg for ₹300) so farmers test it and see results firsthand. Pair with testimonials: "Farmer Y doubled income despite minor feather issues."
- **Outcome:** Sales rise 25% as farmers prioritize their want (profit) over usefulness (perfect health), proving utility drives demand regardless of ethical debates.

9. Form Utility: Transforming Dairy By products into Profit

Question

You're a dairy entrepreneur with excess whey (a byproduct of cheese-making) that farmers dump due to low perceived utility. How can you create form utility to turn whey into a marketable product for the livestock sector, and what steps would you take to convince buyers?

Answer

Form utility comes from reshaping goods—turn whey into a valuable livestock feed supplement.

- **Strategy:** Process whey into a protein-rich powder (e.g., ₹50/kg vs. liquid whey's ₹5/kg disposal cost). Market it as "WheyBoost" for poultry and dairy: "20% more protein than maize at half the cost."
- **Convincing Buyers:** Demonstrate ROI: "Add WheyBoost to feed, gain 10% more milk/eggs in 60 days." Offer free 10kg samples (possession utility) to prove results.
- **Execution:** Partner with a local processor (₹20,000 setup) and sell in 25kg bags, targeting poultry farmers needing cheap protein.

- **Outcome:** Whey shifts from waste to ₹1L monthly revenue, as form utility meets farmers' need for affordable nutrition.

10. Place & Time Utility: Optimizing Veterinary Medicine Distribution

Question

You're a vet supplier with antibiotics that poultry farmers need during disease outbreaks, but rural stock runs out fast, and urban warehouses are too far. How can you use place and time utility to ensure availability and increase sales during peak demand periods?

Answer

Place utility moves goods where they're valued; time utility ensures they're ready when needed.

- **Strategy:** Set up mini-warehouses in rural hubs (e.g., ₹10,000/month rent) stocked with antibiotics (₹50,000 inventory). Use time utility by pre-stocking 20% extra before monsoon outbreaks (peak disease season).
- **Execution:** Offer a "Rush Delivery" service (₹100 fee) from rural hubs, guaranteeing 24-hour access. Promote: "Medicines where and when you need them—save your flock."
- **Outcome:** Sales jump 30% during outbreaks, as place utility (local access) and time utility (timely supply) meet farmers' urgent wants, outpacing urban competitors.

11. Possession Utility: Scaling Dairy Equipment Adoption

Question

You manufacture milking machines (₹25,000 each) that boost dairy efficiency, but small farmers can't afford them and see no utility without ownership. How can you leverage possession utility to get machines into their hands and grow your customer base?

Answer

Possession utility transfers goods to those who value them—make ownership accessible.

- **Strategy:** Launch Ascendancy Leasing Plan: Offer a "Rent-to-Own" model—farmers pay ₹1,000/month for 25 months, then own the machine outright. Start with a ₹2,000 deposit (low entry barrier).
- **Utility Pitch:** Emphasize: "Double your milking speed, save 2 hours daily—yours for ₹33/day." Pair with a free first-month trial (possession utility kickstart).

- **Execution:** Partner with dairy co-ops to manage payments and repossess defaults. Train farmers on-site to ensure they experience efficiency gains.
- **Outcome:** 50 farmers join in 6 months, boosting your sales (₹50,000 revenue/month) as possession utility turns skeptics into owners.

12. Utility and Value Addition in Dairy Farming

Question

Ramesh, a dairy farmer, sells raw milk at Rs. 40 per liter in his village. A local entrepreneur suggests processing the milk into paneer and yogurt, which could be sold at Rs. 250 per kg and Rs. 80 per liter, respectively, in urban markets. How does this strategy enhance the utility of milk, and what type(s) of utility does it create?

Answer

By processing milk into paneer and yogurt, Ramesh creates **form utility**, as the milk is transformed into more valuable products. Additionally, selling these products in urban markets creates **place utility**, where demand is higher. Storing excess products for peak demand times would also generate **time utility**. These strategies can significantly increase Ramesh's income and market reach.

13. Time Utility in Veterinary Services

Question

Dr. Priya, a veterinarian, operates a mobile veterinary clinic in a remote village. She notices that many livestock farmers require vaccinations and deworming services before the monsoon season when disease outbreaks are common. How can she apply the concept of time utility to improve livestock health and increase her service uptake?

Answer

Dr. Priya can create **time utility** by stockpiling vaccines and dewormers before the monsoon season and launching an awareness campaign about their benefits. By offering pre-monsoon vaccination camps, she ensures that farmers get preventive healthcare services at the right time, reducing disease outbreaks and increasing demand for her services.

14. Place Utility in Poultry Farming

Question

Sandeep owns a poultry farm in a rural area, where the local demand for eggs is low, and prices are only Rs. 5 per egg. However, in nearby cities, eggs sell for Rs. 8 each. What steps should Sandeep take to leverage place utility, and how can this decision impact his profits?

Answer

Sandeep can enhance **place utility** by transporting his eggs to urban markets where demand is higher. He can partner with local retailers, grocery stores, or direct-to-consumer delivery services to ensure a steady supply. By selling eggs at Rs. 8 instead of Rs. 5, his revenue increases significantly, improving profitability.

15. Utility and Transferability of Veterinary Equipment

Question

A veterinary entrepreneur, Akash, has surplus veterinary equipment, including AI kits and ultrasound machines. He realizes that many rural veterinary clinics lack these tools but have a demand for them. How can Akash generate possession utility, and what business model can he adopt to maximize returns?

Answer

Akash can create **possession utility** by selling or leasing the equipment to rural veterinary clinics that need it. A **rental or leasing model** can be an effective business approach, allowing rural vets to access expensive equipment without a high upfront cost while ensuring continuous income for Akash.

16. Consumer vs. Capital Goods in Dairy Business

Question

Meera runs a dairy processing unit and wants to invest in either a bulk milk chiller or flavored milk production equipment. The chiller will help store milk longer, while flavored milk production will create a new revenue stream. Based on the concepts of consumer goods and capital goods, which investment should she prioritize for long-term business sustainability?

Answer

The **bulk milk chiller** is a **capital good** as it helps in the production process by preserving milk, reducing spoilage, and ensuring consistent supply. **Flavored milk production** involves consumer goods that provide immediate satisfaction. For long-term sustainability, Meera should first invest in the bulk milk chiller to strengthen her supply chain before expanding into flavored milk, which can enhance her revenue later.

17. Value in Use vs. Value in Exchange: Boosting Poultry Feed Sales

Question

You're a poultry feed entrepreneur selling a premium feed (₹50/kg) with high nutritional value. Farmers value its use (better egg production) but hesitate to buy due to its low exchange value compared to cheaper alternatives (₹40/kg). How can you enhance its perceived value in exchange without lowering the price?

Answer

Value in exchange reflects what farmers are willing to trade for your feed—boost it by tying utility to tangible gains.

- **Strategy:** Bundle the feed with a free egg yield tracker app (worth ₹500) that logs output improvements (e.g., "+10 eggs/week per flock"). Pitch: "Pay ₹50/kg, gain ₹1,000 extra monthly revenue."
- **Execution:** Highlight value in use: "Our feed's nutrition cuts grow-out time by 5 days." Offer a trade-in program—farmers exchange 10 empty premium feed bags for a 5kg bonus bag, increasing exchange appeal.
- **Outcome:** Farmers see ₹50/kg as a fair trade for higher profits and perks, lifting sales by 20% without price cuts, as exchange value aligns with utility.

18. Price and Market Conditions: Competing in Dairy Equipment

Question

You manufacture milking machines priced at ₹25,000, but a competitor slashes their price to ₹20,000 due to lower production costs. Demand shifts to them, despite your machine's superior durability. How can you adjust your pricing strategy, considering supply, demand, and market conditions, to regain market share?

Answer

Price reflects market dynamics—counter competition by emphasizing value over cost.

- **Strategy:** Keep ₹25,000 price but introduce a "Durability Guarantee": free repairs for 3 years (competitor offers 1 year). Add a financing option: ₹5,000 down, ₹500/month for 40 months.
- **Market Play:** Leverage scarcity—limit stock to 50 units/season, creating urgency: "Only 50 left—built to last." Highlight demand: "Top dairies choose us for 20% higher uptime."

- **Outcome:** Sales rebound 15% as farmers prioritize long-term savings (₹10,000 over 5 years) over initial price, shifting demand back despite market competition.

19. Wealth and Income: Scaling a Veterinary Clinic

Question

You run a veterinary clinic with wealth in physical assets (equipment worth ₹5L) and skills (non-salable expertise). Your monthly income is ₹50,000 from consultations, but you want to grow. How can you use your wealth to generate more income without selling assets?

Answer

Wealth generates income—leverage your assets and skills to expand revenue streams.

- **Strategy:** Use equipment for a "Mobile Vet Unit"—offer on-farm services (e.g., ₹1,000/visit) using your tools. Train staff (your skill as wealth) to run a parallel clinic, doubling capacity.
- **Execution:** Invest ₹50,000 from savings into a used van for mobility. Charge ₹500 extra for rural visits, tapping unmet demand. Staff clinic earns ₹30,000/month from urban clients.
- **Outcome:** Income rises to ₹90,000/month (₹40,000 mobile + ₹50,000 clinic), as physical wealth (equipment) and skills amplify earnings without asset sales.

20. Savings and Investment: Expanding a Dairy Farm

Question

You're a dairy farmer earning ₹1L/month from milk sales, with consumption at ₹60,000 (feed, labor). You save ₹40,000 monthly but want to double milk output. How can you convert savings into investment to grow, and what specific assets should you target?

Answer

Savings (Income - Consumption) fuel investment—channel them into productive capital.

- **Strategy:** Invest ₹2L (5 months' savings) in 5 high-yield cows (₹40,000 each). Add ₹50,000 for a fodder chopper to cut feed costs by 10%.
- **Execution:** Cows boost output from 300L to 600L/month (₹50/L = ₹3L revenue). Chopper saves ₹6,000/month on feed, enhancing ROI. Reinvest profits to scale further.

- **Outcome:** Income jumps to ₹2.4L/month (₹3L - ₹60,000 costs), as savings turn into wealth (livestock, machinery), doubling production in 6 months.

21. Consumption and Value: Optimizing Poultry Farm Efficiency

Question

You're a poultry entrepreneur spending ₹2L/month on feed (indirect consumption) to produce 5,000 eggs (final consumption value ₹5/egg). Wasteful consumption (e.g., spoilage) eats 10% of feed. How can you reduce wasteful consumption and increase value for your customers?

Answer

Consumption drives value—cut waste to boost efficiency and customer worth.

- **Strategy:** Install a ₹50,000 feed storage silo to prevent spoilage (10% loss = ₹20,000/month). Market eggs as "FreshMax" at ₹5.5/egg, emphasizing quality from better feed use.
- **Execution:** Train staff on portion control, reducing overfeeding by 5% (₹10,000 saved). Pitch to buyers: "Fresher eggs, higher nutrition—worth the extra ₹0.5."
- **Outcome:** Costs drop to ₹1.7L (₹2L - ₹30,000 savings), revenue rises to ₹2.75L (5,000 x ₹5.5), increasing value in exchange and profit by ₹55,000/month.

22. Unlimited Wants: Expanding a Poultry Feed Business

Question

You're a poultry feed entrepreneur selling a basic feed (₹40/kg) that satisfies farmers' necessaries of existence (bird survival). As farmers' incomes rise, they express new wants for premium feed to boost egg production. How can you capitalize on the unlimited nature of wants to grow your business?

Answer

Wants are endless—once basic needs are met, farmers seek efficiency and comfort.

- **Strategy:** Launch a "Premium EggBoost Feed" (₹50/kg) with added vitamins for 15% higher egg output. Market it as a necessary of efficiency: "Grow more, earn more."
- **Execution:** Offer a free 10kg sample with 100kg basic feed purchases, showing results (e.g., "+5 eggs/bird/week"). Use ads: "Upgrade your flock's potential."

- **Outcome:** 30% of customers shift to premium, lifting revenue from ₹4L to ₹5.5L/month, as new wants for productivity replace basic survival needs.

23. Wants Vary in Urgency: Prioritizing Veterinary Services

Question

You're a veterinarian serving dairy farmers. A mastitis outbreak spikes demand for urgent treatment (₹1,000/cow), but some farmers also want long-term herd health plans (₹5,000/year). How can you address varying urgency and intensity of wants to maximize revenue during the crisis?

Answer

Urgent wants trump future ones—focus on immediate needs while planting seeds for later.

- **Strategy:** Prioritize mastitis treatment with a "Rapid Response Package" (₹1,200 includes medicine + follow-up), meeting the urgent want. Bundle a discounted health plan (₹4,000/year) for post-crisis care.
- **Execution:** Deploy mobile units for same-day service, advertising: "Save your cow today, secure her tomorrow." Train staff to upsell plans during visits.
- **Outcome:** Treat 50 cows/month (₹60,000) and sell 20 plans (₹80,000), totaling ₹1.4L revenue, balancing urgent and future wants.

24. Complementary Wants: Bundling Dairy Equipment

Question

You sell milking machines (₹25,000) to dairy farmers, but sales lag because farmers lack complementary goods like milk cans (₹2,000) to fully utilize them. How can you leverage complementary wants to boost machine sales?

Answer

Wants are complementary—satisfy them together for higher uptake.

- **Strategy:** Bundle a milking machine with a free milk can set (₹2,000 value) as a "Dairy Efficiency Kit" for ₹25,000. Pitch: "Milk faster, store smarter."
- **Execution:** Demo the combo: "Cut milking time by 50%, keep milk fresh for ₹5/L more." Offer financing (₹2,000/month) to ease purchasing power concerns.
- **Outcome:** Sales rise 25% (50 units/month = ₹12.5L), as complementary goods fulfill the want for a complete milking solution.

25. Economic vs. Non-Economic Wants: Innovating Poultry Health

Question

You're a poultry entrepreneur noticing farmers want healthier flocks (economic want) but also desire free advice from vets (non-economic want). How can you turn the non-economic want into an economic opportunity to grow your business?

Answer

Convert non-economic wants into payable services by adding value.

- **Strategy:** Launch a "Flock Care Subscription" (₹500/month) with weekly vet tips via SMS and one free on-farm visit quarterly. Market: "Expert advice, healthier birds."
- **Execution:** Partner with vets to provide tips (₹10,000/month cost), targeting 100 subscribers. Upsell feed or vaccines during visits, meeting economic wants.
- **Outcome:** Earn ₹50,000/month from subscriptions, plus ₹20,000 from upsells, turning free advice into a ₹70,000 revenue stream.

4

Theory of Demand

Definition of Demand

Demand refers to the desire for a commodity that is backed by both purchasing power and willingness to pay at a given price within a specific period. In economics, we consider *effective demand*—not just absolute desire. A product is in demand only when individuals are willing and able to purchase it.

> **Demand**
>
> Demand isn't just wanting something—it's wanting it *and* being able to pay for it at a specific price and time. In economics, this is called **effective demand**. If someone desires a product but can't or won't buy it, it doesn't count
>
> **Key Elements**
>
> - Desire: You want the product.
> - Purchasing Power: You have the money.
> - Willingness to Pay: You're ready to spend.
> - Time Frame: It's specific (e.g., this month).

For example, many farmers may *desire* to buy cow mats, but if they lack the financial resources or are unwilling to spend on them, it does not count as effective demand.

Demand is formally defined as a "schedule or curve that shows the various quantities of a commodity that consumers are willing and able to purchase at different prices, within a specific time frame and market conditions."

Law of Demand

The Law of Demand states that, *ceteris paribus* (all other factors remaining constant), the quantity demanded of a commodity varies inversely with its price. In simpler terms:

When the price of a commodity rises, the quantity demanded decreases. When the price of a commodity falls, the quantity demanded increases.

This inverse relationship occurs because consumers tend to buy less of an expensive product and more of a cheaper one, provided other factors like income, preferences, and the price of related goods remain unchanged.

Examples of the Law of Demand

1. **Milk Price Increase**: If the price of milk increases from ₹60/liter to ₹100/liter, some consumers may reduce their consumption or switch to alternatives like soy milk.
2. **Concentrated Cattle Feed Price:** If the price of concentrated cattle feed rises from Rs 600/bag to Rs 800/bag. Farmers may shift to grazing or cheaper hay. Demand decreases as price rises.

Types of Demand

1. **Price Demand**: Price Demand shows how much of a product people will buy at different prices, assuming everything else (income, tastes, prices of other goods) stays the same. It's the classic demand we see in the Law of Demand—price goes up, quantity demanded goes down; price goes down, quantity demanded goes up.

Price Demand helps you predict how price changes affect sales. For farmers, it's about milk or egg sales; for vets, it's about service bookings.

Example in Vet/Animal Husbandry

- **Milk Pricing**
  i. At Rs 60/liter, consumers buy 1,000 liters/month from a dairy farmer.
  ii. Price rises to Rs 100/liter, demand drops to 600 liters/month—some switch to soy milk or cut back.
  iii. Price falls to Rs 50/liter, demand jumps to 1,200 liters/month—more people stock up.
- **Vet Services**
  i. A vet charges Rs 500 for a cow check-up, and 20 farmers book appointments monthly.
  ii. At Rs 800, only 10 farmers call; at Rs 300, 30 farmers sign up.

2. **Income Demand**: Income demand refers to the various quantities of a commodity that consumers purchase at different levels of income, while the prices of related goods and consumer preferences remain unchanged. Income demand shows how much of a product people buy as their income changes, assuming the product's price and other factors (like tastes) stay constant. When income rises, people often buy more or better goods; when it falls, they cut back or switch to cheaper options. Income demand affects what you can afford to buy (e.g., feed, tools) and what your customers buy from you (e.g., milk). Higher income often means demand for quality goods.

Example in Vet/Animal Husbandry

- **Dairy Farmer's Purchases**
- Income rises from Rs 50,000/month to Rs 80,000/month (good milk sales).
  - Farmer buys premium cattle feed (20 bags at Rs 700/bag) instead of basic feed (30 bags at Rs 400/bag).
  - Might invest Rs 50,000 in an automatic milking machine.
- Income drops to Rs 30,000/month (low sales).
  - Switches to cheaper feed (40 bags at Rs 300/bag) and skips equipment upgrades.
- **Consumer Side**
  - A farmer's family earns more, so they buy 10 litres/week of milk instead of 5 litres/week.
  - If income falls, they drop to 3 litres/week or use powdered milk.

3. **Cross Demand**: Cross demand refers to the quantity of a good that consumers purchase at different prices of a related good, assuming that consumer income and the price of the good itself remain constant. This is relevant for substitutes (e.g., tea and coffee) and complements (e.g., cars and fuel). Cross Demand shows how the demand for one good changes when the price of a *related* good changes, assuming income and the price of the original good stay the same. It applies to:
   - **Substitutes:** Goods that replace each other.
   - **Complements:** Goods used together.

Examples in Vet/Animal Husbandry

i. Substitute Goods

- **Buffalo Milk vs. Cow Milk**
  - Buffalo milk price rises from Rs 70/liter to Rs 90/liter.
  - Demand for cow milk (stable at Rs 60/liter) increases from 800 liters/month to 1,000 liters/month as consumers switch.
  - If buffalo milk drops to Rs 50/liter, cow milk demand might fall to 600 liters/month.
- **Feed Options**
  - Price of concentrated feed jumps from Rs 600/bag to Rs 800/bag.
  - Farmers buy more hay (Rs 400/bag), increasing its demand from 10 tons to 15 tons/month.

ii. Complementary Goods

- **Cattle Fodder and Dairy Cows**
  - Fodder price falls from Rs 10/kg to Rs 5/kg.
  - Farmers buy more fodder (200 kg to 400 kg/month) and increase demand for dairy cows (from 10 to 15 cows) to produce more milk.
  - If fodder price rises to Rs 15/kg, demand for cows might drop as farming becomes less profitable.
- **Vet Services and Livestock**
  - Vaccine prices drop from Rs 200/dose to Rs 100/dose.
  - Farmers vaccinate more goats, boosting demand for vet visits (from 20 to 30 /month)

Autonomous and Derived demand

1. **Autonomous Demand:** Autonomous demand refers to the demand for goods that is **independent** of the demand for other goods. These goods are purchased for their **own sake**, not because they are used to produce something else.

   Examples

   i. **Milk, eggs, and meat** – Consumers buy these for direct consumption.

   ii. **Mobile phones** – People buy them for personal use, not as an input for other goods.

   iii. **Electricity for household use** – Consumers use it for lighting, cooking, and entertainment, independent of industrial demand.

2. **Derived Demand**

   Definition: Derived demand refers to the demand for goods that **depends on the demand for other goods**. These are typically inputs required to produce other goods.

Examples

i. **Livestock** – Farmers rear cows and goats because of the demand for **milk, meat, and wool**.

ii. **Animal feed** – The demand for cattle feed increases with the rising demand for dairy and poultry products.

iii. **Cotton** – The demand for cotton depends on the textile industry's demand for fabric production.

iv. **Construction materials** – Cement and bricks have derived demand as they are needed for real estate and infrastructure projects.

Demand Schedule

A demand schedule is a tabular representation that shows different prices of a commodity, and the corresponding quantities consumers are willing to buy over a specific period.

There are **two types** of demand schedules:

1. **Individual Demand Schedule** – Represents the demand of a **single consumer** at different price levels.
2. **Market Demand Schedule** – Represents the **total demand** of all consumers in the market at different price levels.

Table: Individual Demand Schedule

Price (₹/Liter)	Quantity Demanded per Week (Liters)
70	4
65	5
60	7
55	9
50	11
45	12
40	15

The table shows that as the price decreases, the quantity demanded increases, demonstrating the Law of Demand—consumers demand less at higher prices and more at lower prices.

Table: Market Demand Schedule

(Example: Milk Demand from Four Households in a Town)

The market demand schedule is obtained by summing up the demand from multiple households.

Price of Milk (₹ per liter)	Household A Demand (L)	Household B Demand (L)	Household C Demand (L)	Household D Demand (L)	Total Market Demand (L)
100	1	2	1	2	6
50	3	5	3	4	15
40	5	8	6	7	26
30	8	12	9	10	39
20	12	15	14	16	57
10	18	22	20	24	84

This table shows that **as milk prices decrease, the total market demand increases**, following the **Law of Demand**.

Consumer demand less at higher prices & demand when prices fall. Thus, law of demand guides consumer behavior.

Demand Curve

A demand schedule is converted into d**emand curve** by graphically plotting various **price-quantity combinations.** When the demand schedule is plotted on a graph, with **price on the Y-axis** and **quantity demanded on the X-axis,** we obtain **a demand curve.**

A typical demand curve slopes downwards from left to right, indicating an **inverse relationship between price and quantity demanded**—as the **price decreases, quantity demanded increases,** and vice versa.

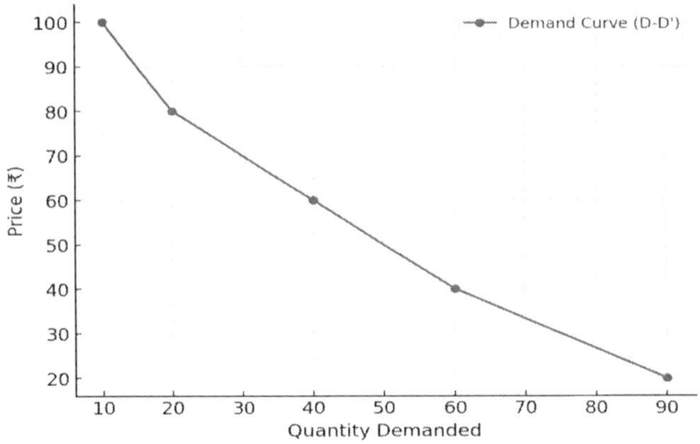

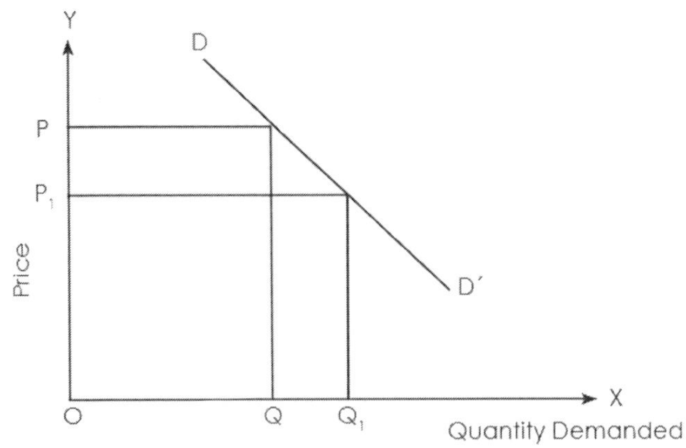

Why does a demand curve slopes downwards? (Reasons for law of demand)

The inverse price-demand relationship is the foundation of the law of Demand**, which states that** when the price of a commodity increases, its quantity demanded decreases, and vice versa, assuming all other factors remain constant. The demand curve slopes downward due to the following key reasons, which explain the Law of Demand:

1. *Income Effect*

i. When the **price of a commodity falls**, the **purchasing power (real income)** of consumers **increases**.

ii. This means they can **buy more of the commodity** even if their actual income remains unchanged.

Example: If the price of **milk** falls from ₹60 to ₹50 per litre, a dairy farmer's family may start consuming more milk or milk-based products like curd and paneer. A dairy farmer's family, with an Rs 300 weekly budget for dairy products, can now buy 6 litres instead of 5. They might use the extra for curd or paneer—demand rises from 5L to 6L due to increased real income. Conversely, if the **price increases**, the real income **decreases**, and consumers **buy less**. For example feed prices jump from Rs 500/bag to Rs 600/bag. With an Rs 5,000 budget, a farmer buys 8 bags instead of 10—real income drops, so demand falls.

2. *Substitution Effect*

i. When the **price of a commodity falls**, it becomes **relatively cheaper** than substitutes, leading consumers to **switch to the cheaper option**.

Example: If the price of **poultry meat** drops from Rs 200/kg to Rs 150/kg; mutton stays at Rs 300/kg. Consumers switch to chicken—demand rises from 50 kg to 70 kg/week. If poultry rises to Rs 250/kg, mutton looks better—chicken demand drops. The price of conventional dewormer rises from Rs 200/dose to Rs 300/dose; herbal dewormer stays at Rs 150/dose. Farmers switch to herbal—demand for conventional dewormer falls, herbal demand rises.

3. Law of Diminishing Marginal Utility

i. As consumers **consume more units** of a product, the **additional satisfaction (marginal utility)** derived from each extra unit **decreases**.

ii. To encourage further consumption, the **price must fall**.

iii. In other words marginal utility is the extra satisfaction from one more unit of a product. The more you consume, the less each additional unit matters—satisfaction fades. To keep buying more, the price must drop to match that lower utility.

iv. **Example:** A household consuming **2 litres milk daily** may not want to buy more unless the price is **reduced**.
   - 2 litres/week = vital (tea, kids).
   - 8 litres/week = less exciting (waste, boredom).
   - They'll only buy 8 if price falls from Rs 60/liter to Rs 40/liter.

The substitution effect is generally stronger and more certain than the income effect because:

1 It always influences consumer choices—when a commodity's price falls, it becomes relatively cheaper than alternatives, prompting consumers to buy more of it.
2. It applies to all types of goods—whether normal, superior, or inferior, consumers will prefer the cheaper option if substitutes exist.
   - **Downward Slope:** Price down = demand up, thanks to:
     - **Income Effect:** More buying power.
     - **Substitution Effect:** Cheaper wins over substitutes.
     - **Diminishing Utility:** Extra units need lower prices.

Effects of Price Change on Different Types of Goods

The way demand shifts when prices change depends on the type of good. The **Income Effect** (change in purchasing power) and **Substitution Effect** (switching to cheaper options) drive these shifts, but their impact varies between **Normal/Superior Goods** and **Inferior Goods**.

1. Normal or Superior Goods

1. **Examples:** Milk, meat, eggs, herbal veterinary products.
2. These are goods people want more of as their income rises (normal) or high-quality versions they prefer when they can afford them (superior).
3. For **normal and superior goods**, the **income effect** and **substitution effect** work in the **same direction.**
4. **How Price Changes Work:**

   Price Falls

   i. Income Effect: Real income rises—you feel richer and can buy more of the good.

   ii. Substitution Effect: It's cheaper than alternatives, so you switch to it.

   iii. Result: Both effects push demand *up*—they work together.

Price Rises

i. **Income Effect:** Real income shrinks—you feel poorer and buy less.

ii. **Substitution Effect:** Alternatives look cheaper, so you switch away.

iii. **Result:** Both effects push demand *down*.

Example

i. If **pasteurized milk** price drops, consumers **buy more pasteurized milk** instead of raw milk.

ii. If **herbal veterinary medicine** becomes cheaper, dairy farmers **shift from chemical-based treatments**.

For normal/superior goods, price cuts boost demand doubly (income + substitution), while price hikes cut it hard. Farmers and vets see this with premium products like organic milk or herbal treatments.

2. Inferior Goods

1. These are lower-quality goods people buy when income is tight but ditch for better options when they can afford it.
2. **How Price Changes Work:**

Price Falls

- **Substitution Effect:** It's cheaper than alternatives, so people buy more.
- **Income Effect:** Real income rises, but people might switch to better goods instead.
- **Result:** Substitution usually wins, so demand rises slightly—opposing effects clash.

Price Rises

- **Substitution Effect:** Alternatives get relatively cheaper, so people switch away.
- **Income Effect:** Real income falls, pushing people back to the inferior good.
- **Result:** Demand might not drop much—or could rise—since income effect counters substitution.

Example

i. If the price of **maize or broken rice (used in poultry feed)** increases, some **small farmers may buy more maize** instead of switching to costly alternatives like **soya meal**.

ii. If the price of **low-cost veterinary medicines** increases, some **farmers may still buy them** instead of **shifting to expensive branded products**.

Exceptions to the Law of Demand

In some special cases, demand for a commodity increases even when its price rises, which contradicts the usual inverse relationship between price and demand. These exceptions occur due to various social, psychological, and economic reasons.

1. Giffen's Goods (Giffen's Paradox)

i. These are inferior goods (cheap, low-quality staples) where demand rises when their price increases because the income effect outweighs the substitution effect. Poor consumers can't afford better options, so they stick with the inferior good even as it gets pricier.

ii. Named after Robert Giffen, who observed that when the price of bread increased, low-paid British workers bought more bread instead of switching to other foods.

iii. Example in Animal Husbandry: Poor farmers relying on bajra (pearl millet) for feeding cattle may buy more bajra if its price rises because they cannot afford costlier alternatives like commercial cattle feed or soya meal.

2. Conspicuous Goods (Veblen Goods)

i. Luxury goods where demand increases with price because they signal status and prestige. Higher prices make them more desirable to wealthy buyers.

ii. Price rises → perceived value or exclusivity grows → demand increases.

iii. Named after Thorstein Veblen, who introduced the concept of "conspicuous consumption."

iv. Examples in Animal Husbandry:

a) Thoroughbred/Arabian Racehorses

a) Price jumps from Rs 5 lakh to Rs 7 lakh per horse.

b) Elite owners buy more (e.g., 2 to 3 horses) to flaunt wealth at races—high price = high status.

b) A2 Milk Cows (Gir, Sahiwal)

a) Price rises from Rs 50,000 to Rs 70,000 per cow.

b) Dairy farmers or boutique farms demand more (e.g., 5 to 7 cows) because premium pricing signals quality and exclusivity for A2 milk markets.

v. For vets or farmers in premium markets, high prices can attract buyers who want to stand out—think organic or niche livestock.

3. Speculation Effect

Demand rises with price when people expect prices to climb even higher in the future. They buy now to avoid shortages or bigger costs later.

Reason

- Price rises → fear of worse prices or scarcity → stock up now.

Examples in Animal Husbandry

Cattle Feed Shortage

i. Feed price rises from Rs 500/bag to Rs 600/bag amid drought rumors.

ii. Farmers buy more (e.g., 20 bags to 30 bags/month) to hoard before it hits Rs 800/bag or runs out.

Chick Prices Before Festivals

i. Chick price jumps from Rs 30 to Rs 40 due to festival demand speculation.

ii. Poultry farmers stock up (e.g., 1,000 to 1,500 chicks) expecting Rs 50/chick soon.

Key Insight

Farmers and vets see this during supply scares—panic buying defies the usual "price up, demand down" rule.

4. Bandwagon Effect (Social Influence on Demand)

1. Demand rises with price when social trends, peer pressure, or promotion push people to follow the crowd—regardless of cost.
2. **Reason:**Price rises → popularity or hype grows → demand increases.
3. **Examples in Animal Husbandry**

   a) **Gir/Sahiwal Cows:** Price rises from Rs 50,000 to Rs 70,000 due to government subsidies or progressive farmer buzz.

   More farmers buy (e.g., 10 to 15 cows in a region) to join the trend, even at a premium.

   b) **Herbal Veterinary Medicines:** Price jumps from Rs 150/dose to Rs 200/dose after social media raves.

   Dairy farmers switch (e.g., 20 to 30 doses/month) because "everyone's doing it."

Key Insight

Social pressure can override price logic—vets and farmers tap into trends (e.g., organic, native breeds) to boost demand.

Key Takeaways

- **Exceptions Exist:** Demand can rise with price in rare cases.
- **Reasons:** Poverty (Giffen), prestige/quality (Veblen), fear (speculation), or trends (bandwagon).
- Normal Curve: Downward (price up = demand down).
- Exceptions: Upward slope (price up = demand up).
  - i. **Giffen:** Income traps poor buyers.
  - ii. **Veblen:** Status/quality drives rich buyers.
  - iii. **Speculation:** Fear fuels hoarding.
  - iv. **Bandwagon:** Trends pull everyone in.

Extension and Contraction of Demand vs. Increase and Decrease in Demand

Extension and Contraction of Demand

i. These are changes in the **quantity demanded** caused *only* by a change in the price of the good, with all other factors (income, tastes, etc.) held constant. They are movements *along the same demand curve.*

ii. **Extension of Demand:** When the **price of a good falls**, its **quantity demanded increases** (movement **down along the demand curve**).

iii. **Contraction of Demand:** When the **price of a good rises**, its **quantity demanded decreases** (movement **up along the demand curve**).

Examples

i. **Milk Price Drops from ₹60 to ₹40 per Litre:** More consumers buy milk → **Extension of Demand.**

ii. **Broiler Chicken Price Increases from ₹200 to ₹250/kg:** Consumers shift to tofu or other protein sources → **Contraction of Demand.**

Graphically

i. **Downward movement from A to B** = **Extension of Demand** (due to price decrease).

ii. **Upward movement from B to A** = **Contraction of Demand** (due to price increase).

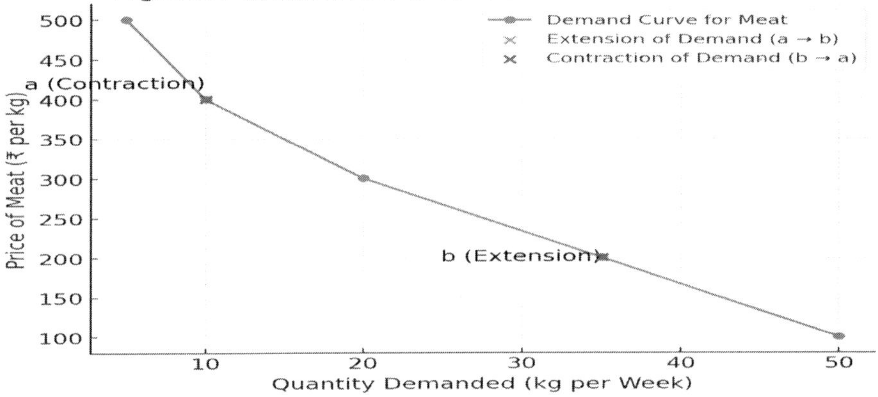

Fig.1.5: Extension and Contraction of Demand

3. Increase and Decrease in Demand

i. These are changes in demand itself caused by factors *other than price* (e.g., income, tastes, prices of related goods). The entire demand curve shifts:

ii. Increase in Demand**:** More demanded at the same price → curve shifts *right.*

iii. Decrease in Demand**:** Less demanded at the same price → curve shifts *left.*

Factors Influencing Demand Shifts

Increase in Demand

i. Rising **disposable income** increases milk & dairy product consumption.

ii. **Dietary preferences** shifting towards **protein-rich dairy**.

iii. **Government initiatives** like the **Mid-Day Meal Scheme** increasing milk demand.

iv. **Festivals (Diwali, Navratri, etc.)** boosting demand for **ghee, curd, and sweets**.

v. **Fast-food chains (McDonald's, KFC, Domino's)** increasing demand for **processed chicken products**.

Decrease in Demand

i. **Lumpy Skin Disease (LSD) outbreak** causing a **fear-driven decline** in milk consumption.

ii. **Rise of veganism & plant-based alternatives** reducing milk demand, especially in **urban centers**.

iii. **Avian influenza outbreaks** leading to **temporary boycotts of chicken**.

iv. **Religious observances (Shravan, Navami, etc.)** lowering poultry & egg consumption.

Graphically

i. **Rightward shift = Increase in Demand**.

ii. **Leftward shift = Decrease in Demand**.

Difference between Extension/Contraction and Increase/Decrease in Demand

Concept	Definition	Example in Animal Husbandry
Extension of Demand	Quantity demanded increases due to fall in price of the good (movement down the same demand curve).	If milk price falls from ₹60 to ₹40 per liter, more people buy milk.
Contraction of Demand	Quantity demanded decreases due to rise in price of the good (movement up the same demand curve).	If broiler chicken price rises from ₹200 to ₹250/kg, consumers switch to tofu or other protein sources.
Increase in Demand	Demand curve shifts right due to non-price factors like higher income, trend changes, or government policies.	If more consumers start preferring farm-fresh organic milk, demand increases even if price remains same.
Decrease in Demand	Demand curve shifts left due to non-price factors like lower income, change in preferences, or availability of substitutes.	If synthetic meat or plant-based milk alternatives become popular, demand for traditional milk may decrease.

Factors Affecting Demand (Determinants of Demand)

These factors change demand at the *same price*, unlike price changes that move you along the curve (extension/contraction). These are known as **shift factors**. When they shift demand, the whole curve moves—right for an increase, left for a decrease.

1. Income of the Consumer

How much money people have affects what they buy. More income usually means more demand for better goods; less income can shift demand to cheaper options.

- **Normal Goods:** Demand rises with income.
- **Inferior Goods:** Demand falls as income rises (people upgrade).

Examples in Vet/Animal Husbandry

Normal Goods

Pet owners' income rises from Rs 50,000 to Rs 80,000/month.

Demand for premium pet accessories (e.g., organic treats, fancy collars) jumps from 10 units to 20 units/month at Rs 500 each.

Inferior Goods

Small dairy farmers' income increases from Rs 20,000 to Rs 40,000/month.

Demand for broken maize (cheap feed) drops from 100 kg to 50 kg/month at Rs 15/kg, as they switch to premium cattle feed (Rs 30/kg).

2. Consumer's Taste and Preferences

What people like or value shifts demand. Trends, habits, or cultural shifts can make a product hot or not.

Examples in Vet/Animal Husbandry

Veganism Trend

- Rising veganism boosts plant-based milk demand (e.g., soy milk) from 50L to 100L/week at Rs 60/liter, while cow milk demand softens.

Festival Demand

- During Bakrid, demand for goat meat spikes from 200 kg to 500 kg/week at Rs 600/kg due to cultural preference.

3. Size and Composition of Population

More people = more demand. The age or type of population also tweaks what's in demand.

Examples in Vet/Animal Husbandry

Population Growth

A town's population grows from 10,000 to 15,000.

Demand for milk, meat, and eggs rises (e.g., milk from 10,000L to 15,000L/month at Rs 60/litre).

Age Composition

Young families increase → milk demand jumps (e.g., 5L to 7L/week per household at Rs 50/litre).

Elderly population grows → demand shifts to low-fat dairy (e.g., 2L to 4L/week at Rs 70/litre).

4. *Change in Fashion & Weather*

Seasons or trends shift what people want—weather especially hits food and farm products.

Examples in Vet/Animal Husbandry

Cold Weather

Demand for ghee and butter rises from 50 kg to 80 kg/month at Rs 500/kg—warm, rich foods rule winter.

Hot Weather

Curd and buttermilk demand jumps from 100L to 150L/week at Rs 40/liter—cooling options for summer.

5. Price of Related Goods

i. **Substitute Goods:** If the price of **chicken** rises, demand for **fish or plant-based meat alternatives** may increase.
ii. **Complementary Goods:** If the price of **paneer falls**, demand for **spices and vegetables for paneer dishes** may increase.

6. Change in Quantity of Money in Circulation

More money floating around (e.g., economic boom) boosts purchasing power, lifting demand for premium goods.

Example

Economic Boom

i. Money supply grows—farmers and consumers have more cash.
ii. Demand for A2 milk rises from 50L to 80L/week at Rs 100/liter; organic eggs jump from 1,000 to 1,500/month at Rs 10 each.

7. Technological Progress

Better tech (e.g., processing, packaging) makes goods more appealing or accessible, boosting demand.

Examples in Vet/Animal Husbandry

Dairy Tech

i. New packaging extends milk shelf life.
ii. Demand for processed milk rises from 5,000L to 7,000L/month at Rs 60/liter—convenience wins.

Vet Tools

i. Portable ultrasound devices improve diagnostics.

ii. Demand for vet services jumps from 20 to 30 visits/month at Rs 500/visit.

8. *Advertisement and Promotions*

Marketing or campaigns sway consumer behavior, shifting demand up (or down if negative).

Examples in Vet/Animal Husbandry

Fast-Food Ads

i. KFC/McDonald's push chicken nuggets.

ii. Demand for processed chicken rises from 500 kg to 800 kg/week at Rs 300/kg.

Government Campaigns

i. Mid-Day Meal Scheme promotes milk.

ii. School milk demand jumps from 1,000L to 1,500L/month at Rs 50/liter.

Elasticity & Its Importance in Policy and Business Decision-Making

Elasticity is a key economic concept that helps policymakers and businesses analyze how sensitive demand is Vto changes in price, income, or related goods.

Types of Elasticity

1. **Price Elasticity of Demand (PED)**: Measures how much demand changes when price changes.

   Example: If the price of milk rises from ₹50 to ₹60 per liter, will people still buy the same amount, or will demand drop?

2. **Income Elasticity of Demand (YED)**: Measures how demand changes with income levels.

   Example: If rural incomes rise, will more people shift to A2 milk or organic dairy products?

3. **Cross-Price Elasticity of Demand (XED)**: Measures how demand for one product changes when the price of another related product changes. Example: If chicken prices rise, will consumers switch to eggs or plant-based proteins instead?

Why Is Elasticity Important for Policymakers and Businesses?

i. *Government Policies and Subsidies* – Helps decide taxation, subsidies, and minimum support prices for dairy, poultry, and livestock sectors.

ii. *Dairy and Poultry Industry Decisions* – Helps set optimal prices for milk, eggs, and meat based on demand response.

iii. *Livestock Farming and Feed Costing* – Predicts how farmers will react to changes in fodder, feed, and medicine prices.

Types of Price Elasticity of Demand (PED) with Examples in Dairy, Animal Husbandry and Veterinary Sectors

1. **Perfectly Elastic Demand (ed = ∞):** A small decrease in price leads to an infinite increase in demand.

   Example: If a milk supplier sells pasteurized milk at ₹50 per liter, but another offers it at ₹49 per liter, consumers will shift entirely to the lower-priced supplier. Graph: The demand curve is a horizontal straight line (parallel to X-axis).

2. **Relatively Elastic Demand (ed> 1)**: The percentage change in demand is more than the percentage change in price.

   Example: Luxury dairy products like organic milk, A2 cow milk, and exotic cheese are price-sensitive. A 10 percent drop in price could lead to a 30 percent rise in demand. Graph: The demand curve is flatter, showing a larger increase in demand compared to price change.

3. **Unit Elastic Demand (ed = 1)**: The percentage change in demand is equal to the percentage change in price.Example: Animal vaccines or medicines – If a deworming drug price increases by 15 percent, its demand may also decrease by 15 percent, as farmers have fixed seasonal vaccination plans. Graph: The demand curve is a rectangular hyperbola.

4. **Relatively Inelastic Demand (ed< 1)**: The percentage change in demand is less than the percentage change in price.

   Example: Dairy milk for household consumption – If milk prices increase by 20 percent, demand may only drop by 5 percent, as it is a daily necessity. Graph: The demand curve is steeper, indicating smaller demand changes.

5. **Perfectly Inelastic Demand (ed = 0)**: Demand remains constant, no matter how much the price changes.

   Example: Life-saving animal medicines and vaccines – Farmers will buy essential vaccines for cattle regardless of price to prevent disease outbreaks. Graph: The demand curve is a vertical straight line.

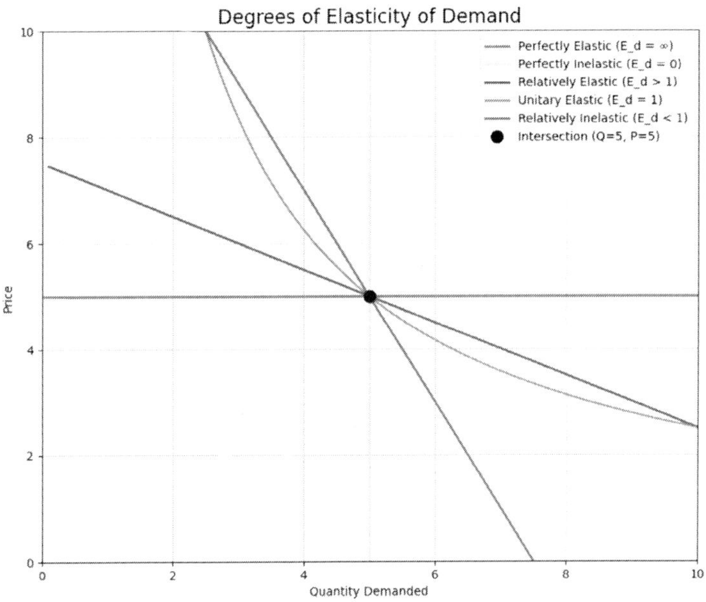

Understanding price elasticity helps: Dairy and Poultry Farmers adjust prices to maximize sales. Veterinarians and Feed Suppliers predict demand fluctuations. Policymakers set subsidies and taxation policies for livestock farmers.

Income elasticity of demand

It is ratio of proportionate change in quantity demanded resulting from a proportionate change in income.

$$\text{Income Elasticity of Demand} = \frac{\%\text{ change in quantity demanded}}{\%\text{ change in income}}$$

Based on values of income elasticity, we can classify goods as luxuries, necessities and inferior goods.

1. Luxury – A goods is said to "luxury", if its income elasticity is greater than one. As income rises, consumers spend a larger proportion of their income on these goods. For eexample: Premium pet grooming services or specialized veterinary treatments, Organic Dairy Product
2. Necessity - A commodity is necessity, if its income elasticity is small (less than one as income increases, quantity demanded rises, but the proportion of income spent on these goods decreases. For example basic veterinary care (e.g., vaccinations, deworming) or standard livestock feed, normal milk and eggs

3. Inferior - A commodity is inferior if the income elasticity is negative. Low-quality animal feed (e.g., cheap, unbranded grain mixes).

Distinction between Necessities and Inferior Goods

For necessities, an increase in income leads to an increase in quantity demanded, but it becomes a smaller part of the budget (less proportional spending).

For inferior goods, an increase in income causes an absolute decline in demand as consumers opt for better substitutes.

Cross elasticity of demand

1. Cross elasticity of demand measures how the quantity demanded of one good responds to a change in the price of another good
2. Proportionate change in the quantity demanded of a good resulting from a proportionate change in the price of a related good.

Complimentary goods

i. Cross elasticity is negative.
ii. As the price of one good increases, demand for both goods falls.
iii. Example: Tea and sugar, car and petrol.

Substitute Goods

i. Cross elasticity is positive.
ii. An increase in the price of one good leads to an increase in demand for its substitute.
iii. Example: Chicken and mutton.

Income Elasticity of Demand
1. **Luxury Goods**: Income elasticity > 1
2. **Necessities**: Income elasticity < 1 (but positive)
3. **Inferior Goods**: Income elasticity < 0 (negative)
Cross elasticity of demand
1. **Complementary Goods:** Cross elasticity < 0 (negative)
2. **Substitute Goods:** Cross elasticity > 0 (positive)
Few Examples

Analytical Questions

1. Law of Demand: Pricing veterinary services during a disease outbreak

Question

You're a veterinarian charging ₹500 per farm visit for poultry health checks. A disease outbreak increases demand, but raising your fee to ₹800 reduces bookings from 50 to 30 per month. How can you use the Law of Demand to optimize pricing and maximize revenue during the crisis?

Answer

The Law of Demand shows an inverse price-quantity relationship—adjust pricing to balance demand and income.

1. **Strategy:** Set a tiered pricing model: ₹500 for basic checkups (50 visits/month) and ₹700 for an "Outbreak Special" (checkup + vaccine, targeting 20 visits). Total revenue: (50 x ₹500) + (20 x ₹700) = ₹39,000 vs. ₹40,000 at ₹800 (30 visits).
2. **Execution:** Promote: "Basic care at ₹500, full protection at ₹700—save your flock." Offer a 10% discount on the first 10 Outbreak Special bookings to boost uptake.
3. **Outcome:** Bookings rise to 70/month (50 basic + 20 special), revenue hits ₹39,000, leveraging the Law of Demand to capture more demand at lower prices.

2. Price Demand: adjusting dairy product sales?

Question

You're a dairy farmer selling milk at ₹60/liter, with 1,000 liters/month demand. A competitor drops their price to ₹50/liter, and your sales fall to 800 liters. How can you use price demand principles to regain market share without matching their price?

Answer

Price demand shows quantity falls as price rises—enhance value to maintain demand.

- **Strategy:** Keep ₹60/liter but add value: bundle 10 liters with a free 500ml yogurt (₹20 value). Pitch: "Premium milk + bonus yogurt—worth ₹80 for ₹60."
- **Execution:** Target loyal customers with a "Milk Plus" subscription (10L/week, ₹600, yogurt included). Advertise quality: "Rich taste, higher nutrition."
- **Outcome:** Sales rebound to 1,100 liters/month (₹66,000 vs. ₹48,000 at competitor's rate), as perceived value offsets price sensitivity, per price demand dynamics.

3. Price Demand in Dairy Farming

Question

A dairy farmer named Ramesh has been selling milk at ₹60 per liter, with a daily demand of 100 liters. Due to increased production costs, he raises the price to ₹80 per liter. However, his sales drop to 70 liters per day. What economic principle is observed here, and what should Ramesh consider to maintain profitability?

Answer

This is an example of **Price Demand**, following the **Law of Demand**, which states that as the price of a commodity increases, demand decreases (ceteris paribus). Ramesh should consider:

1. Offering incentives (e.g., discounts for bulk buyers).
2. Improving milk quality to justify higher prices.
3. Exploring alternative revenue sources like paneer or ghee production.

4. Pricing Strategy for a Vet Clinic

Question

Dr. Sneha runs a veterinary clinic. She raises consultation fees from ₹400 to ₹700 per visit, but her monthly bookings drop from 50 to 30. What should she consider to optimize revenue?

Answer

This follows the **Law of Demand**—higher prices lead to lower demand. Dr. Sneha can:

1. Introduce loyalty programs or package deals.
2. Offer teleconsultations at lower rates.
3. Differentiate by providing premium services at higher prices.

5. Income Demand: Upselling Poultry Feed as Incomes Rise

Question

You sell basic poultry feed (₹400/bag, 50 bags/month) to farmers earning ₹50,000/month. A bumper harvest boosts their income to ₹80,000/month, and they start eyeing premium feed (₹600/bag). How can you use income demand to shift them to higher-value products?

Answer

Income demand rises with income—capitalize on their ability to pay more.

- **Strategy:** Introduce a "Growth Max Feed" (₹600/bag) with 20% higher protein: "More eggs, bigger birds." Offer a transition deal: buy 10 basic bags, get 1 Growth Max free.

- **Execution:** Host field days showing results: "Farmers using Growth Max earn ₹5,000 extra/month." Push financing (₹200/month/bag) to ease the jump.
- **Outcome:** 30 farmers switch (30 x ₹600 = ₹18,000) while 20 stay basic (20 x ₹400 = ₹8,000), totalling ₹26,000/month, tapping income demand growth.

6. Income Demand for Veterinary Services

Question

Dr. Ankit, a veterinary practitioner, notices that when farmers' income rises, they request more preventive healthcare services (vaccination, deworming). When income falls, they only call him in emergencies. How does income demand affect his business strategy?

Answer

Dr. Ankit observes **Income Demand**, where higher income leads to increased demand for quality services. To address this:

1. Offer flexible payment plans for preventive care.
2. Educate farmers on cost-saving benefits of regular check-ups.
3. Introduce tiered service plans to cater to different income groups.

7. Income Demand in a Dairy Business

Question

Arun, a dairy entrepreneur, notices that when local incomes rise, customers switch to premium organic milk, but when incomes fall, they buy regular milk or powdered milk. How should he adjust his product strategy?

Answer

This is **Income Demand**. Arun should:

1. Offer a range of products to cater to different income levels.
2. Market premium milk as a health investment rather than a luxury.
3. Introduce smaller pack sizes of organic milk for budget-conscious consumers.

8. Cross Demand: Competing with Substitutes in Dairy Feed

Question

You sell concentrated cattle feed (₹600/bag, 40 bags/month) to dairy farmers. A hay supplier cuts prices from ₹400 to ₹300/bag, and your sales drop to 25 bags as farmers switch substitutes. How can you use cross demand to regain sales?

Answer

Cross demand shifts with related goods' prices—counter substitutes with differentiation.

- **Strategy:** Position your feed as superior: "20% more milk vs. hay alone." Offer a combo: 5 bags (₹600) + 1 free vet checkup (₹500 value), undercutting hay's appeal.
- **Execution:** Advertise: "Hay saves ₹100 now, our feed earns ₹1,000 later." Target 10 lost customers with a 10% discount (₹540/bag) for 3 months.
- **Outcome:** Sales recover to 35 bags/month (₹21,000), as cross demand shifts back—farmers value milk yield over hay's short-term savings.

9. Cross Demand in Poultry Farming

Question

A poultry farmer, Priya, notices that when soybean meal (a key poultry feed ingredient) becomes expensive, farmers shift to maize-based feed. What concept does this illustrate, and how should Priya plan her business?

Answer

This is **Cross Demand** involving **substitute goods** (soybean meal vs. maize). Priya can:

1. Stock alternative feed options based on price trends.
2. Blend feeds to optimize costs without reducing nutrition.
3. Monitor market trends and advise fellow farmers.

10. Cross Demand between Buffalo and Cow Milk

Question

A restaurant chain primarily uses buffalo milk but switches to cow milk when buffalo milk prices rise. How can a dairy supplier stabilize demand?

Answer

This is **Cross Demand** between **substitutes** (buffalo vs. cow milk). The supplier can:

1. Offer blended milk options (mixing buffalo and cow milk).
2. Educate customers about the nutritional benefits of both types.
3. Lock in bulk buyers with fixed-price contracts.

11. Derived Demand in Dairy Farming

Question

A rural entrepreneur, Sunil, sells cattle feed. He notices that when milk prices rise, farmers buy more feed, but when milk prices drop, feed sales decline. Why does this happen, and how can Sunil manage demand fluctuations?

Answer

This is an example of **Derived Demand**—feed demand depends on milk demand. Sunil can:

1. Diversify into related products like fodder or mineral supplements.
2. Offer credit schemes to retain customers during low-price periods.
3. Develop bundled offers (e.g., discounts for bulk feed purchases).

12. Autonomous Demand for Eggs

Question

A supermarket reports that even during economic downturns, egg sales remain stable. What type of demand does this represent, and how can poultry entrepreneurs leverage this?

Answer

This is **Autonomous Demand**—eggs are essential food items, so demand remains stable. Poultry entrepreneurs should:

1. Focus on consistent supply and quality.
2. Differentiate products (organic eggs, fortified eggs).
3. Expand to new customer segments (e.g., bakeries, hotels).

13. Individual Demand Schedule: Pricing Veterinary Consultations

Question

You're a veterinarian charging ₹500 per consultation, with a farmer demanding 5 visits/month. Your individual demand schedule shows: ₹600 (3 visits), ₹500 (5 visits), ₹400 (7 visits), ₹300 (10 visits). How can you use this schedule to set a price that maximizes revenue while keeping the farmer engaged?

Answer

An individual demand schedule maps one consumer's response—optimize revenue within it.

- **Analysis:**
  - ₹600: 3 visits = ₹1,800
  - ₹500: 5 visits = ₹2,500
  - ₹400: 7 visits = ₹2,800
  - ₹300: 10 visits = ₹3,000
- **Strategy:** Set price at ₹300/visit to maximize revenue (₹3,000). Boost engagement with a "Health Pass": 10 visits at ₹300 each, prepaid, with a free vaccine (₹200 value).
- **Execution:** Pitch: "Full care at ₹300/visit—save your flock and your wallet." Use the downward slope (more visits at lower prices) to lock in commitment.
- **Outcome:** Farmer buys 10 visits (₹3,000 vs. ₹2,500 at ₹500), increasing revenue by 20% via the schedule's insights.

14. Market Demand Schedule: Scaling Milk Sales in a Village

Question

You're a dairy farmer with a market demand schedule for milk: ₹50/L (15L/week), ₹40/L (26L/week), ₹30/L (39L/week) across four households. A rival offers milk at ₹45/L, cutting your sales to 20L at ₹50/L. How can you use the market schedule to adjust pricing and regain demand?

Answer

A market demand schedule sums total demand—use it to outmanoeuvre competition.

- **Strategy:** Drop price to ₹40/L (26L/week demand) and add value: free 250ml milk with every 5L. Pitch: "More milk for less than ₹45/L."
- **Execution:** Promote: "₹40/L beats ₹45/L—stock up now." Target 30L/week by offering a 5% discount (₹38/L) for bulk (10L+) buyers, pushing past 26L.
- **Outcome:** Sales hit 30L/week (₹1,200 vs. ₹900 at ₹45/L rival rate), as the downward curve drives higher demand at a competitive price.

15. Demand Curve: Launching Poultry Feed Variants

Question

You sell poultry feed at ₹600/bag, with 20 bags/month demand. Your demand curve data shows: ₹700 (15 bags), ₹600 (20 bags), ₹500 (25 bags), ₹400 (30 bags). Farmers resist higher prices due to cheaper alternatives. How can you use the demand curve to introduce a new variant and boost sales?

Answer

The demand curve's downward slope guides pricing—offer options to capture more demand.

- **Strategy:** Launch a "Lite Feed" at ₹400/bag (30 bags demand) alongside premium at ₹600 (20 bags). Total revenue: (30 x ₹400) + (20 x ₹600) = ₹24,000 vs. ₹12,000 at ₹600 alone.
- **Execution:** Market Lite as "Affordable Nutrition" and premium as "Max Growth." Offer a free 5kg sample of Lite with 10 premium bags to cross-sell.
- **Outcome:** Sales rise to 50 bags/month (₹24,000), doubling revenue by leveraging the curve's price-quantity trade-off.

16. Individual Demand Schedule: Selling Dairy Equipment

Question

You sell milking machines with an individual demand schedule for a farmer: ₹30,000 (1 unit), ₹25,000 (2 units), ₹20,000 (3 units). At ₹30,000, they buy 1, but you want to sell more. How can you use this schedule to encourage bulk purchases?

Answer

An individual schedule shows willingness—lower prices to spur more buys.

- **Strategy:** Price at ₹20,000/unit for 3 units (₹60,000 revenue vs. ₹30,000 for 1 at ₹30,000). Sweeten with free installation (₹2,000 value): "Triple efficiency, one price."
- **Execution:** Demo: "3 machines = 30L/hour vs. 10L—worth ₹5,000/month." Offer a 6-month payment plan (₹10,000 upfront, ₹8,333/month).
- **Outcome:** Farmer buys 3 units (₹60,000), tripling revenue as the downward slope incentivizes bulk demand.

17. Market Demand Curve: Competing in Egg Sales

Question

You sell eggs with a market demand schedule: ₹6/egg (100 eggs/week), ₹5/egg (150 eggs), ₹4/egg (200 eggs) across a town. A competitor prices at ₹5.50/egg, dropping your sales from 150 to 120 at ₹5. How can you use the demand curve to regain market share?

Answer

The market demand curve slopes down—adjust price and value to pull demand back.

- **Strategy:** Set price at ₹4/egg (200 eggs/week, ₹800) and bundle: 10 eggs + free recipe card (₹10 value). Pitch: "Cheaper, tastier eggs."
- **Execution:** Advertise: "₹4/egg beats ₹5.50—feed your family more." Target 20% above 200 eggs (240 eggs) with a loyalty deal: buy 50 eggs, get 5 free.
- **Outcome:** Sales hit 220 eggs/week (₹880 vs. ₹660 at ₹5.50 rival rate), as the curve's lower price drives higher market demand.

18. Impact of Price Reduction on Milk Sales

Question

A dairy entrepreneur notices that when the price of milk drops from ₹60 to ₹50 per liter, families buy more milk and milk-based products. Why does this happen, and how can the entrepreneur use this insight for business growth?

Answer

This follows the **Income Effect**, where a lower price increases the consumer's purchasing power, allowing them to buy more. The entrepreneur can use this insight by offering bulk discounts or launching **value-added dairy products** (curd, paneer) to capture the increased demand.

19. Substitutes in Veterinary Medicine

Question

A veterinarian sells a conventional dewormer at ₹300/dose. When a herbal dewormer at ₹150/dose enters the market, farmers switch to the herbal option. How does this relate to the Law of Demand?

Answer

This is the Substitution Effect—farmers choose the cheaper herbal alternative. The veterinarian can respond by offering promotions on the conventional dewormer or emphasizing its superior effectiveness to retain customers.

20. Declining Demand for Poultry Feed

Question

A poultry farmer budgets ₹5,000 for feed each month. If feed prices increase from ₹500 to ₹600 per bag, how will this affect his purchasing behavior?

Answer

Due to the Income Effect, the farmer's purchasing power decreases—he can now buy only 8 bags instead of 10. To manage this, he may:

1. Reduce the number of birds to lower feed costs.
2. Seek alternative feeds or bulk purchase discounts.
3. Raise chicken prices to offset feed cost increases.

21. Substitution effect in meat consumption

Question

If poultry prices drop from ₹200/kg to ₹150/kg while mutton remains at ₹300/kg, how will consumer behavior shift?

Answer

Consumers will switch to the **cheaper poultry meat**, increasing demand. Poultry farmers can use this opportunity to:

- Promote chicken as a **cheaper, healthier alternative**.
- Offer **special cuts or processed poultry** to further attract customers.

22. Selling more dairy products through pricing

Question

A dairy farmer sells 2 liters of milk per household daily at ₹60/liter. Families hesitate to buy more, but when the price drops to ₹40/liter, weekly purchases increase to 8 liters. What economic principle explains this?

Answer

This follows the Law of Diminishing Marginal Utility—consumers value extra units less, so a price drop encourages higher consumption. The farmer can introduce bulk purchase incentives (e.g., "Buy 5 liters, get 1 free") to boost sales.

23. Income Effect: Expanding Milk Sales to Farmers' Families

Question

You're a dairy farmer selling milk at ₹60/liter, with a family buying 5 liters/week on a ₹300 budget. When you drop the price to ₹50/liter, they only increase to 6 liters. How can you amplify the income effect to boost their demand further?

Answer

The income effect increases real income when prices fall—highlight extra purchasing power.

- **Strategy:** Drop to ₹50/liter and bundle: 10 liters + free 500ml curd (₹20 value) for ₹500. Pitch: "More milk, more meals—same budget."
- **Execution:** Show savings: "₹60 saved (from ₹60/L) buys 1L extra + curd." Promote uses: "Make paneer, feed kids." Offer a 5% loyalty discount (₹47.5/L) for 10L+ weekly.
- **Outcome:** Demand rises to 10 liters/week (₹500 vs. ₹300 at ₹60/L), as the income effect (₹60 extra real income) drives higher consumption.

24. Substitution Effect: Competing in Poultry Feed Markets

Question

You sell poultry feed at ₹600/bag, with 30 bags/month demand. A rival drops hay prices from ₹400 to ₹350/bag, cutting your sales to 20 bags. How can you use the substitution effect to regain demand without lowering your price below ₹600?

Answer

The substitution effect favors cheaper options—make your feed the better choice.

- **Strategy:** Keep ₹600/bag but enhance value: 10 bags + free vitamin pack (₹100 value). Pitch: "20% more eggs vs. hay's 5%—worth ₹600."
- **Execution:** Advertise: "Hay's cheap, our feed's profitable—switch back." Demo results: "Farmer X gained ₹2,000/month with our feed."
- **Outcome:** Sales rebound to 35 bags/month (₹21,000), as the substitution effect shifts demand from hay to your superior feed.

25. Diminishing Marginal Utility: Selling Bulk Veterinary Vaccines

Question

You sell poultry vaccines at ₹200/dose, with a farmer buying 10 doses/month for a 100-bird flock. At ₹150/dose, they buy 15 doses, but resist more due to lower utility. How can you use diminishing marginal utility to encourage bulk purchases?

Answer

Diminishing marginal utility reduces extra satisfaction—lower prices and add value for more units.

- **Strategy:** Offer 20 doses at ₹120/dose (₹2,400 total) with free delivery (₹200 value). Pitch: "Full flock protection, lower cost per bird."
- **Execution:** Explain: "10 doses = 80% coverage, 20 doses = 100%—worth it at ₹120." Target larger flocks with a trial (5 doses at ₹150).

- **Outcome:** Farmer buys 20 doses (₹2,400 vs. ₹2,000 at ₹200), as lower price offsets utility drop, boosting sales by 20%.

26. Income and Substitution Effects: Positioning Dairy Equipment

Question

You sell milking machines at ₹25,000, with 10 units/month demand. A hand-milking tool drops from ₹5,000 to ₹4,000, cutting your sales to 7 units. How can you use income and substitution effects to regain demand?

Answer

Income and substitution effects drive the curve—enhance affordability and value.

- **Strategy:** Keep ₹25,000 but offer a "Dairy Boost Kit": machine + free milk can (₹2,000 value). Pitch: "Save ₹5,000/year vs. hand tools."
- **Execution:** Promote income effect: "₹25,000 = 20L/day, ₹10,000 extra income." Substitution effect: "Faster than ₹4,000 tools, better milk quality." Add a ₹5,000 down payment plan (₹1,667/month).
- **Outcome:** Sales rise to 12 units/month (₹3L), as income (more profit) and substitution (beats hand tools) effects pull demand back.

27. All Three Effects: Optimizing Egg Sales

Question

You sell eggs at ₹6/egg, with 100 eggs/week demand. A rival drops to ₹5/egg, cutting your sales to 80 eggs. How can you use income effect, substitution effect, and diminishing marginal utility to adjust pricing and regain market share?

Answer

All three effects shape the downward slope—combine them for impact.

- **Strategy:** Drop to ₹4.5/egg (target 150 eggs/week) with a "Family Pack": 20 eggs + free recipe (₹10 value). Pitch: "Cheaper, tastier, more eggs."
- **Execution**
  - **Income Effect:** "₹1.5/egg saved = 3 extra eggs free in your ₹90 budget."
  - **Substitution Effect:** "₹4.5 beats ₹5—switch to us."
  - **Diminishing Utility:** "20 eggs at ₹4.5 = meals all week, worth it." Promote via local shops.

- **Outcome:** Sales hit 160 eggs/week (₹720 vs. ₹400 at ₹5 rival rate), as all effects drive higher demand down the curve.

28. Speculation and Bandwagon Effects: Selling Chicks Pre-Festival

Question

You sell chicks at ₹30 each, with 1,000/month demand. Festival rumors push prices to ₹40, and demand jumps to 1,500 due to speculation and hype. How can you use speculation and bandwagon effects to maximize sales?

Answer

Speculation (fear of higher prices) and bandwagon (trend-following) defy the downward slope.

- **Strategy:** Raise to ₹40/chick and pitch: "Stock up now—prices may hit ₹50." Bundle 100 chicks + free feed sample (₹100 value) for ₹4,000.
- **Execution**
    - **Speculation:** "Festival rush—buy before shortages."
    - **Bandwagon:** "Top farmers are stocking up—join them." Advertise via WhatsApp groups and local markets.
- **Outcome:** Sales hit 2,000 chicks/month (₹80,000 vs. ₹30,000 at ₹30), as speculation (hoarding) and bandwagon (hype) fuel an upward demand surge.

29. Giffen Goods in Cattle Feed

Case: In a remote village, bajra (pearl millet) is the primary cattle feed. If the price of bajra increases, will farmers buy less or more of it?

Answer

Unlike normal goods, demand for bajra may increase despite the price hike. Poor farmers, unable to afford better alternatives like commercial feed, might allocate more of their budget to bajra, making it a Giffen good.

30. Veblen Effect in Livestock Trading

Case: A dairy farm offers Gir cows at a higher price, marketing them as premium A2 milk producers. Instead of reducing demand, the price increase leads to higher sales. Why?

Answer

This is an example of the **Veblen Effect**. Wealthier dairy farmers perceive expensive Gir cows as superior and prestigious. The higher price signals exclusivity and quality, leading to an increase in demand.

31. Speculation Effect in Poultry Business

Case: Rumors suggest that chick prices will increase from ₹30 to ₹50 per chick in the coming months. What will poultry farmers do?

Answer

Farmers may buy and stock up on chicks now to avoid paying a higher price later. This speculation effect causes current demand to rise due to expectations of future price hikes.

32. Bandwagon Effect in Veterinary Products

Case: A new herbal veterinary supplement gains popularity through social media endorsements. Its price rises from ₹150 to ₹200 per dose, but demand keeps increasing. Why?

Answer

The **Bandwagon Effect** is at play. Farmers see others switching to the herbal supplement and follow the trend, even though it is more expensive.

33. Effect of Price Change on Superior Dairy Products

Case: A dairy cooperative introduces organic, grass-fed butter. Initially priced at ₹500/kg, the price increases to ₹700/kg. Yet, demand increases. Why?

Answer

Organic butter falls under the **Veblen Goods category**. Wealthier consumers associate the higher price with better quality and exclusivity, leading to higher demand.

34. Impact of Feed Price Rise on Small Dairy Farmers

Case: Due to supply shortages, cattle feed prices rise from ₹500 to ₹700 per bag. How will small dairy farmers react?

Answer

Small farmers may:

- Reduce feed quantity per animal.
- Switch to lower-cost alternatives (e.g., maize, husk).
- Increase grazing to offset feed costs.
- In extreme cases, sell off less productive animals. This response depends on the balance between the **income effect** (less purchasing power) and the **substitution effect** (switching to alternatives).

35. Price Change and Demand Shifts in Dairy Farming

Case: A dairy farmer producing A2 milk notices that its price has risen from ₹50 to ₹70 per liter due to increasing awareness of its health benefits. Despite the price hike, demand continues to grow.

Question

Which economic principle explains this phenomenon, and how should the farmer respond to maximize profit?

Answer

This is an example of the **Veblen Effect**, where higher prices signal superior quality and exclusivity, leading to increased demand. The farmer can capitalize on this trend by branding A2 milk as a premium product, marketing its health benefits, and expanding sales to niche urban markets.

36. Speculation Effect in Poultry Farming

Case: A poultry farmer observes that due to an upcoming festival season, the price of broiler chicks is increasing from ₹30 to ₹40. Expecting further hikes, many farmers start stocking more chicks.

Question

What economic effect is at play here, and what risk does it carry?

Answer

This is the **Speculation Effect**, where farmers buy more due to expectations of even higher prices. However, the risk is that if demand does not materialize as expected, oversupply could lead to price crashes post-festival, causing losses. Entrepreneurs should monitor market trends and avoid excessive stocking.

37. Inferior Goods and Small Farmers' Choices

Case: A small-scale dairy farmer usually buys low-cost mineral mixtures for cattle. When its price increases, instead of switching to a superior product, he continues buying the same or even more.

Question

Why does the farmer behave this way, and which economic principle applies?

Answer

This behavior is explained by **Giffen's Paradox**—the farmer, constrained by budget, cannot afford superior alternatives and ends up buying more of the inferior good despite its price rise. To assist such farmers, policymakers can introduce subsidies or bulk-purchase schemes for quality feed.

38. Bandwagon Effect in Veterinary Medicine

Case: A new herbal veterinary medicine for mastitis gains popularity on social media. Even after its price rises from ₹150 to ₹200 per dose, more dairy farmers start using it.

Question

Which economic principle explains this trend, and how can a veterinary entrepreneur leverage it?

Answer

This is the **Bandwagon Effect**, where demand increases due to social influence. A veterinary entrepreneur can take advantage of this by promoting the product through influencer marketing, testimonials from progressive farmers, and social media campaigns to sustain demand.

39. Extension vs. Increase in Demand in Cattle Feed

Case: A drought leads to higher prices for commercial cattle feed. Farmers reduce their feed purchases and switch to alternative sources like farm-grown fodder.

Question

Is this an example of contraction of demand or a decrease in demand? Why?

Answer

This is **contraction of demand**, as it results from a price increase leading to lower quantity demanded (movement up along the same demand curve). A decrease in demand, in contrast, would occur if farmers permanently shifted to alternative feeds due to changing preferences or innovations.

40. Dairy Farmer's Pricing Dilemma

Question

Rajesh, a dairy farmer in Himachal Pradesh, sells fresh cow milk at ₹60 per liter. Recently, he reduced the price to ₹50 per liter to attract more customers. He noticed a significant rise in daily milk sales.

- *What type of demand change is observed here—extension, contraction, increase, or decrease in demand?*
- *How would this affect his overall revenue?*
- *If the price of dairy-based plant alternatives (like almond milk) drops in the market, how might it impact Rajesh's business?*

Answer

- This is an **Extension of Demand** because the increase in sales is due to a reduction in milk price.
- Whether revenue increases or decreases depends on **elasticity of demand**—if the demand is elastic, revenue will rise; if inelastic, revenue may decline.
- If plant-based alternatives become cheaper, demand for cow milk may **Decrease**, shifting the demand curve left.

41. Broiler Farmer's Challenge with Price Increase

Question

Pooja, a broiler chicken farmer, used to sell chicken at ₹200/kg. Due to rising feed costs, she had to increase the price to ₹250/kg. However, she noticed a drop in customer orders, as many shifted to eggs or plant-based protein.

- *What type of demand change is occurring here?*
- *How can Pooja minimize the negative impact of this contraction?*
- *If a popular fast-food chain starts sourcing more chicken for burgers, what would happen to the demand curve?*

Answer

- This is a **Contraction of Demand** because the drop in quantity demanded is due to a price increase.
- Pooja can **reduce costs** by optimizing feed expenses, offering combo deals, or branding her product as "organic" or "free-range" to justify the higher price.
- If a fast-food chain increases chicken purchases, **Demand will Increase**, shifting the demand curve right.

42. Expansion of Dairy Business During Festivals

Question

During Diwali, Prakash, who runs a dairy business in Kangra, observed a significant rise in demand for paneer, curd, and ghee—even though he kept the prices the same.

- **Is this an extension or an increase in demand? Why?**
- **What strategy should Prakash adopt to maximize profits during festive seasons?**

- **If post-Diwali, demand suddenly drops, what should he do to maintain sales?**

Answer

- This is an **Increase in Demand** because the demand rose due to a **festival** rather than a price change.
- Prakash should **stock more milk**, introduce festive discounts, and **target bulk buyers like sweet shops**.
- Post-Diwali, he can **introduce loyalty discounts**, explore online sales, or diversify into products with longer shelf life, like **flavored milk or packaged dairy sweets**.

43. Impact of Health Concerns on Poultry Demand

Question

Suresh, a poultry entrepreneur, observed that after news of an avian influenza outbreak, his sales of chicken and eggs declined sharply, even though he did not change his prices.

- *Is this a contraction or a decrease in demand? Why?*
- *How can Suresh regain consumer trust and demand?*
- *If the government initiates a campaign promoting poultry as a safe and nutritious protein source, what will happen to demand?*

Answer

- This is a **Decrease in Demand** because fear of avian flu affected consumer preference, shifting the demand curve left.
- Suresh should educate customers on **biosecurity measures, safe poultry handling, and disease-free certification**.
- A government awareness campaign would lead to an **Increase in Demand**, shifting the demand curve right.

44. Organic Milk Market Growth

Question

Anjali started an organic dairy farm and priced her organic milk at ₹80 per liter, compared to regular milk at ₹50. Initially, demand was low, but after extensive marketing about the health benefits, her sales increased significantly.

- *Is this an extension or an increase in demand? Why?*
- *What key factors helped shift the demand curve?*

- *How can Anjali further strengthen her business in the premium dairy market?*

Answer

- This is an **Increase in Demand** because sales increased due to marketing efforts rather than a price drop.
- Factors influencing demand: **health-conscious consumers, social media influence, and premium branding**.
- Anjali can expand by offering **subscription-based home delivery, partnerships with health stores, and value-added products like organic ghee or A2 milk**.

45. Impact of Income on Demand for Premium Pet Products

Question

Ravi, a pet shop owner in Shimla, noticed that his sales of organic pet food and premium accessories increased when a new IT park opened in the city, bringing in high-salaried professionals. However, during an economic downturn, sales of premium products dropped, and pet owners switched to cheaper alternatives.

- *Which determinant of demand is influencing this trend?*
- *How can Ravi adjust his business strategy to sustain revenue during low-income periods?*
- *What type of product (normal or inferior) is premium pet food?*

Answer

- The **income of the consumer** is the key determinant, as higher income increases demand for premium products and lower income shifts demand to cheaper alternatives.
- Ravi should diversify his product range by offering **budget-friendly pet food options** alongside premium ones to cater to different income levels.
- **Premium pet food is a normal good**, as its demand increases with income and decreases when income falls.

46: Consumer Preferences & Demand for Plant-Based Dairy

Question

Meera runs a dairy farm in Delhi and sells traditional cow milk. However, she observed a decline in demand due to an increasing number of consumers shifting to almond and soy milk, influenced by health trends and vegan lifestyles.

- *Which factor is affecting the demand for cow milk?*
- *Is this a case of a substitute good or a complementary good? Why?*
- *How can Meera reposition her business to maintain demand?*

Answer

- The factor affecting demand is **Consumer Taste and Preferences**, as people are shifting towards plant-based alternatives.
- **Almond and soy milk are substitute goods** for cow milk because they serve the same purpose (milk consumption).
- Meera can **reposition her dairy** by branding her milk as **organic, A2 milk, or farm-fresh** to appeal to health-conscious consumers. She could also diversify into **value-added dairy products like probiotic curd, ghee, or paneer**.

47. Impact of Population Growth on Dairy Demand

Question

In a growing town, a local dairy entrepreneur, Harish, noticed that his milk sales increased significantly after several apartment complexes were built nearby, bringing in new families and young children.

- *Which determinant of demand is responsible for this increase?*
- *What strategy should Harish adopt to handle this rise in demand?*
- *How would demand change if a significant number of elderly people moved in instead?*

Answer

- The determinant affecting demand is **Size and Composition of Population**. More families with children increase milk consumption.
- Harish should **scale up milk production**, explore **home delivery services**, and form **bulk supply contracts with apartments**.
- If more elderly people moved in, demand might **shift from full-cream milk to low-fat or skimmed milk**.

48. Seasonal Demand for Dairy Products

Question

Sonia runs a dairy processing unit and observed that during winter, demand for ghee and butter increased, while in summer, buttermilk and curd sales surged.

- *Which determinant of demand is influencing this trend?*
- *What strategy should Sonia adopt to maximize profits in both seasons?*
- *If there is an unseasonal heatwave in winter, what impact will it have on dairy demand?*

Answer

- The factor influencing demand is **Change in Weather & Seasonal Preferences**.
- Sonia should **adjust production and marketing strategies seasonally—stock more butter and ghee in winter** and **focus on curd and buttermilk promotions in summer**.
- An unseasonal heatwave in winter would **reduce demand for butter/ghee and increase demand for cooling products like buttermilk and curd**.

49. Effect of Substitute Goods on Poultry Demand

Question

Amit, a poultry farmer, noticed that when the price of chicken increased from ₹200/kg to ₹250/kg, many customers switched to fish, reducing his sales.

- *What type of goods are chicken and fish in this case?*
- *Which determinant of demand is affecting Amit's sales?*
- *What pricing strategy can Amit adopt to retain customers?*

Answer

- Chicken and fish are **substitute goods**, as they fulfill the same dietary need.
- The determinant affecting demand is **Price of Related Goods (Substitutes)**.
- Amit can introduce **combo deals**, offer **discounts on bulk purchases**, or promote **farm-fresh antibiotic-free chicken** to retain his customer base.

50. Impact of Money Supply on Organic Dairy Products

Question

In an economic boom, urban consumers had higher disposable incomes, leading to a surge in demand for organic A2 milk, despite its high price. However, during an economic slowdown, demand dropped as people switched back to regular milk.

- Which determinant of demand is at play?
- Why did demand change despite the price remaining the same?
- How can an organic dairy farm sustain sales during an economic downturn?

Answer

- The determinant is **Change in Quantity of Money in Circulation**—higher money supply increases purchasing power, boosting demand for premium goods.
- Demand changed because, during an economic slowdown, **people prioritize affordability over premium quality**.
- The organic dairy farm can introduce **loyalty programs, small packaging options (half-liter packs), or subscription discounts** to retain customers.

51. Role of Technology in Expanding Veterinary Services

Question

Dr. Priya, a veterinarian, recently invested in portable ultrasound equipment for livestock diagnostics. After advertising her advanced services, she observed an increase in the number of farmers seeking her services, even though her consultation charges remained unchanged.

- *Which determinant of demand is influencing this increase?*
- *Why did demand rise even though prices didn't change?*
- *How can Dr. Priya further enhance her veterinary practice using technology?*

Answer

- The determinant at play is **Technological Progress**.
- Demand increased because **better technology improves service quality and attracts more customers**.
- Dr. Priya can enhance her practice by **offering telemedicine consultations, AI-based disease prediction, or partnering with dairy cooperatives for preventive health programs**.

52. Impact of Advertisements on Poultry Demand

Question

A popular fast-food chain launched an aggressive ad campaign promoting its crispy chicken burgers. As a result, local poultry farmers saw a sharp rise in demand for broiler chickens from restaurant suppliers.

- *Which determinant of demand is affecting poultry sales?*
- *What would happen to demand if a negative news report linked broiler chicken to health concerns?*
- *How can poultry farmers leverage advertising for long-term benefits?*

Answer

- The determinant of demand is **Advertisement and Promotions**, as ads influence consumer preferences.
- A negative news report could **decrease demand sharply**, shifting the demand curve left.
- Poultry farmers should invest in **branding, highlight farm hygiene, use influencer marketing, and partner with retailers for promotional discounts** to maintain a strong market presence.

53. Income of the Consumer: Upselling Premium Veterinary Products

Question

You're a veterinary supplier selling basic pet vaccines at ₹200/dose, with 50 doses/month demand. Pet owners' incomes rise from ₹50,000 to ₹80,000/month, but demand only increases to 55 doses. How can you use the income factor to shift demand further for premium products?

Answer

Rising income boosts demand for normal goods—push premium offerings.

- **Strategy:** Introduce a "Pet Wellness Pack" (vaccine + organic supplement) at ₹300/dose. Pitch: "Healthier pets with your bigger budget."
- **Execution:** Target 20 high-income owners with a demo: "₹80,000 income = ₹300 care—boost immunity 20%." Offer a 10% discount (₹270/dose) for first 10 buyers.
- **Outcome:** Demand shifts right to 70 doses/month (50 basic at ₹200 + 20 premium at ₹300 = ₹16,000 vs. ₹10,000), as income drives demand for superior goods.

54. Consumer's Taste and Preferences: Capitalizing on Dairy Trends

Question

You sell cow milk at ₹60/liter, with 1,000 liters/month demand. A veganism trend cuts demand to 800 liters, while plant-based milk gains traction. How can you use shifting preferences to increase demand for your dairy products?

Answer

Taste shifts demand—adapt to counter or ride trends.

- **Strategy:** Launch a "Lactose-Free Cow Milk" at ₹70/liter for health-conscious buyers. Pitch: "Dairy taste, vegan-friendly."
- **Execution:** Promote via social media: "Love milk, hate lactose? Try us—beats soy at ₹80/L." Offer a free 500ml sample with 5L purchases to 50 new customers.
- **Outcome:** Demand shifts right to 1,200 liters/month (800 regular at ₹60 + 400 lactose-free at ₹70 = ₹76,000), reversing the veganism-driven decrease.

55. Size and Composition of Population: Expanding Poultry Egg Sales

Question

You sell eggs at ₹5/egg, with 2,000 eggs/month demand in a town of 10,000. Population grows to 15,000, with more young families, but demand only rises to 2,200 eggs. How can you use population growth to shift demand further?

Answer

More people, especially young families, increase demand—target them.

- **Strategy:** Offer a "Family Egg Pack": 30 eggs at ₹4.5/egg (₹135 total). Pitch: "Feed your kids—more eggs, same price."
- **Execution:** Distribute flyers at schools: "Growing town, growing kids—stock up." Add a 10% discount (₹121.50/pack) for 50+ eggs monthly.
- **Outcome:** Demand shifts right to 3,000 eggs/month (₹13,500 vs. ₹11,000), as population size and composition (family focus) boost egg demand.

56. Price of Related Goods: Competing in Poultry Meat Markets

Question

You sell chicken at ₹200/kg, with 500 kg/month demand. Fish prices drop from ₹250/kg to ₹180/kg, cutting your demand to 400 kg. How can you use the price of substitute goods to shift demand back to chicken?

Answer

Substitute price changes shift demand—make chicken more appealing.

- **Strategy:** Keep ₹200/kg and bundle: 5 kg + free spice mix (₹20 value) for ₹1,000. Pitch: "Tastier than fish at ₹180/kg."

- **Execution:** Promote: "Chicken beats fish—₹40/kg meal vs. ₹45." Target 20 fish buyers with a trial (2 kg at ₹190/kg), showing flavor edge.
- **Outcome:** Demand shifts right to 550 kg/month (₹1.1L vs. ₹80,000), as the substitution effect (fish price drop) is countered by chicken's value.

57. Advertisement and Promotions: Boosting Dairy Product Demand

Question

You sell ghee at ₹500/kg, with 50 kg/month demand. A rival's ad campaign lifts their ghee sales, dropping yours to 40 kg. How can you use advertising to shift demand back and grow your market?

Answer

Ads shift demand—outshine competitors with promotion.

- **Strategy:** Keep ₹500/kg and launch a "Pure Ghee Campaign": 1 kg + free recipe booklet (₹30 value). Pitch: "Authentic taste, unbeatable quality."
- **Execution:** Run a social media ad (₹5,000 cost): "Our ghee's the real deal—try it." Partner with 10 local sweet shops for demos, targeting 20 new buyers.
- **Outcome:** Demand shifts right to 70 kg/month (₹35,000 vs. ₹20,000), as advertising reverses the decrease and builds preference.

58. Explain with example why the substitution effect is stronger and more certain than the income effect?

1. Always Kicks In

- Substitution happens every time a price changes relative to alternatives. If poultry drops to Rs 150/kg, people switch from mutton—no hesitation.
- Income effect depends on how much the price change affects your budget. A Rs 10 drop in milk might not feel like a big "raise" if you spend Rs 10,000/month elsewhere.

2. Works for All Goods

- Substitution applies whether it's:
- **Normal goods:** Milk (buy more if cheaper than soy).
- **Superior goods:** Organic feed (switch if cheaper than regular).
- **Inferior goods:** Cheap hay (buy if pricey feed rises).
- Income effect might not boost inferior goods (e.g., cheap feed) when income rises—people upgrade instead.

3. Predictable Impact

- Substitution is a sure bet: cheaper poultry = more poultry demand.
- Income effect varies—Rs 50 vs. Rs 60 milk might not change a rich farmer's habits much, but it could for a poor one.

Example Comparison

- **Poultry Price Drop (Rs 200 to Rs 150):**
- **Substitution:** Everyone switches from mutton—demand spikes.
- **Income:** Some buy more poultry, but if it's a small budget item, the "extra income" might not matter.
- Substitution drives the bigger shift

59. Why income effect, substitution effect and diminishing marginal utility may matter for farmers and Veterinary entrepreneurs?

- **Farmers**
  - **Income Effect:** Cheaper feed means more cows fed—or more profit to spend elsewhere.
  - **Substitution:** High milk prices push buyers to alternatives (soy); low prices keep them loyal.
  - **Utility:** You won't buy extra feed unless it's cheap—cows don't need it past a point.
- **Vets**
  - **Income Effect:** Lower vaccine prices mean farmers can afford more visits.
  - **Substitution:** If your fees rise, farmers might try herbal cures instead.
  - **Utility:** Clients won't pay Rs 500 for a fifth check-up unless it's discounted.

60. How a Poultry Feed Company(NutriFeed Poultry Solutions) used demand principles to Boost Sales?

Background

- **Company:** NutriFeed Poultry Solutions
- **Product:** Protein-rich poultry feed (₹50/kg)
- **Challenge:** Stagnating sales despite strong poultry demand
- **Root Cause:** Competitors offered cheaper feed (₹45/kg), and farmers viewed premium feed as "non-essential"

Answer: NutriFeed Poultry Solutions turned stagnant sales into an 80% growth in six months by applying three key demand principles: the income effect, substitution effect, and diminishing marginal utility. Here's how they did it:

Step 1: Income Effect – Reframing Feed as an Investment

Problem: Farmers saw premium feed as a cost, not a profit driver.

Solution

- Launched an educational campaign with data: "NutriFeed boosts chicken weight gain by 15%, increasing profits."
- Highlighted ROI: Higher income offsets the ₹50/kg price. **Result:** Demand rose 10% as farmers shifted their mindset from expense to earnings.

Step 2: Substitution Effect – Tiered Options to Outmaneuver Rivals

Problem: Farmers opted for cheaper maize mixes (₹35/kg, lower protein).

Solution

- Introduced two products:
- *Premium Feed:* ₹50/kg (high protein)
- *NutriFeed Lite:* ₹40/kg (budget-friendly, decent protein)
- Positioned Lite as a maize alternative, Premium as the profit-maximizer. **Result:** Lite captured price-sensitive buyers; Premium sales grew as farmers upgraded over time.

Step 3: Diminishing Marginal Utility – Bulk Deals to Build Loyalty

Problem: Small, infrequent purchases signaled low commitment.

Solution

- Offered bulk discounts: 5% off 100kg, 12% off 500kg.
- Added a nudge: Free 10kg samples for new buyers (tangible results drove repeats).

  Result: Average order size jumped 30%, locking in bigger sales.

Outcome (6 Months Later)

Metric	Before	After
Monthly Sales	10,000 kg	18,000 kg
Avg. Price/kg	₹50	₹47*
Farmer Retention Rate	40%	75%
**Lower avg. price reflects bulk discounts, but revenue soared from ₹5L to ₹8.46L.*		

Key Demand Principles

1. **Income Effect:** Repositioned feed as a profit booster, not a cost sink.
2. **Substitution Effect:** Tiered pricing stole share from cheap rivals.
3. **Diminishing Utility:** Bulk incentives kept farmers buying more, countering purchase fatigue.

Lessons for Vet & Livestock Businesses

- **Educate:** Link products to income (e.g., "Vaccines = healthier cows = 20% more milk").
- **Tier Up:** Offer premium and budget options to grab every customer segment.
- **Bulk Smart:** Use discounts or bundles (e.g., "Annual parasite control: 15% off") to secure loyalty.
- **Vet Clinic Example:** Bundle "checkup + vaccine" at a discount to beat standalone competitors.
- **Dairy Farm Tactic:** Reward feed purchases with loyalty points for free extras (e.g., mineral supplements).

  By blending economics with farmer psychology, NutriFeed didn't just sell feed—they sold success.

62. Explain with examples in Vet/Animal Husbandry how income and substitution effect work in same direction whenever there is price change for a normal or superior good?

- **Pasteurized Milk**
  - Price drops from Rs 60/liter to Rs 50/liter.
  - **Income Effect:** A family's Rs 300 budget now buys 6 liters instead of 5—more milk for tea or kids.
  - **Substitution Effect:** Cheaper than raw milk (Rs 55/liter), so they switch from raw to pasteurized.
  - **Demand:** Rises from 5L to 7L/week.
  - Price rises to Rs 70/liter:
  - **Income Effect:** Rs 300 buys only 4 liters—less milk consumed.
  - **Substitution Effect:** Raw milk (Rs 55/liter) wins—demand shifts away.
  - **Demand:** Falls to 3L/week.

- **Herbal Veterinary Medicine**
  - Price drops from Rs 200/dose to Rs 150/dose (chemical meds at Rs 250/dose).
  - **Income Effect:** Farmers save Rs 50/dose, affording 10 doses instead of 8 with a Rs 2,000 budget.
  - **Substitution Effect:** Cheaper than chemical meds, so they switch.
  - **Demand:** Jumps from 8 to 12 doses/month.
  - Price rises to Rs 300/dose:
  - **Income Effect:** Rs 2,000 buys only 6 doses—less treatment.
  - **Substitution Effect:** Chemical meds (Rs 250/dose) take over.
  - **Demand:** Drops to 5 doses/month.

63. Income Elasticity (Luxury Goods): Adding Fancy Pet Toys

Question

You sell pet food in a town. People's income goes up, and they want fancy pet toys instead. How can you use luxury goods to sell more?

Answer

Luxury goods are popular when people have more money—sell fun stuff.

- **Strategy:** Start selling pet toys like balls and chew sticks. Say: "Treat your pet like a star!"
- **Execution:** Put toys in your shop and tell richer pet owners: "Spoil your dog!"
- **Outcome:** You sell more toys as people spend extra cash, growing your business.

64. Income Elasticity (Necessity Goods): Keeping Milk Simple

Question

You sell milk to farmers. Their income rises, but they don't buy much more milk. How can you use necessity goods to keep them buying?

Answer

Necessities don't grow much with income—keep it basic and steady.

- **Strategy:** Keep milk prices the same and easy to buy. Say: "Milk you need every day!"
- **Execution:** Offer small packs at your usual price and tell farmers: "Always here for you!"
- **Outcome:** Farmers keep buying milk as a daily need, not a big extra

65. Income Elasticity (Inferior Goods): Switching Cheap Feed

Question

You sell cheap poultry feed to small farmers. Their income goes up, and they stop buying it. How can you use inferior goods to change your plan?

Answer

Inferior goods lose fans when income rises—sell better stuff.

- **Strategy:** Offer a nicer feed for healthier chickens. Say: "Grow strong birds!"
- **Execution:** Stock better feed and tell farmers: "Upgrade your farm!"
- **Outcome:** You sell to farmers who want quality now, not just cheap options.

66. Cross Elasticity (Substitute Goods): Beating Fish with Chicken

Question

You sell chicken meat. Fish prices drop, and people buy fish instead. How can you use substitute goods to bring them back?

Answer

Substitutes compete—make chicken more tempting.

- **Strategy:** Lower your chicken price a little. Say: "Chicken's tastier than fish!"
- **Execution:** Tell buyers: "Special deal on chicken!" and show it's a better choice.
- **Outcome:** People switch back to chicken because it's cheaper and good.

67. Cross Elasticity (Complementary Goods): Pairing Dairy Feed with Milk Buckets

Question

You sell milk buckets to dairy farmers. The price of cow feed goes up, and fewer farmers buy your buckets. How can you use complementary goods to sell more buckets?

Answer

Complements work together—connect buckets to feed.

- **Strategy:** Offer a deal: buy feed and get a discount on buckets. Say: "Feed your cows, fill your buckets!"
- **Execution:** Partner with a feed supplier and tell farmers: "Grab both for less!"

- **Outcome:** Farmers buy your buckets again because they need them with feed, keeping your sales going.

68. As income of rural dairy farmers increases, will they invest more in advanced milking machines or continue with manual methods? Why?

Answer

Manual milking is often a **necessity or even inferior good** compared to **automated milking machines**. As income rises, farmers may shift to mechanization to save time and improve hygiene—indicating that demand for milking machines has a **high positive income elasticity**. Agri-tech businesses should target rising-income rural pockets with cost-effective tech solutions.

5

Utility and The Law of Diminishing Marginal Utility

Definition of Utility

Utility is the ability of a good or service to satisfy human wants and needs in economics. It is an important concept as it represents the satisfaction experienced by a consumer from consuming a good or service

Utility characteristics

1. Measuring satisfaction, benefit, or happiness from a good or service is difficult.
2. Economists have devised ways to represent and measure utility in terms of economic choices that can be quantified.
3. **Total Utility (TU):** The aggregate sum of satisfaction or benefit gained from consuming a given amount of goods or services (e.g., drinking three glasses of water provides more satisfaction than just one).
4. **Marginal Utility (MU):** The additional satisfaction gained from each extra unit of consumption (e.g., the first glass of water gives maximum satisfaction compared to each additional glass).
5. Total utility usually **increases** as more goods are consumed.
6. Marginal utility typically **decreases** with each additional unit consumed, demonstrating the **Law of Diminishing Marginal Utility**.

Law of Diminishing Marginal Utility

1. This law is a fundamental concept in economics that explains consumer behaviour.
2. It states that as an individual consumes more units of a commodity, the marginal utility derived from each successive unit decreases until it becomes zero or negative.
3. Marginal utility is expressed in terms of the price a consumer is willing to pay for a commodity.

4. The law is based on the principle of satiability—each specific want can be satisfied over time.

Illustration of the Law of Diminishing Marginal Utility

1. This law is based on introspection and observation of consumer behavior.
2. While total human wants are unlimited, a single want is satiable.
3. As a consumer consumes more of a good, the intensity of desire for that good declines until a point is reached where additional consumption provides no satisfaction.

Table: Illustration of Diminishing marginal utility

Units of Milk consumed	Total Utility (Utils) derived from the consumption of all units	Marginal Utility (Utils) derived from consumption of every additional units of Milk
1	12	12
2	22	10
3	30	8
4	36	6
5	40	4
6	42	2
7	43	1
8	43	0
9	42	-1
10	40	-2
11	36	-4

Graphical Illustration of Law of Diminishing marginal utility

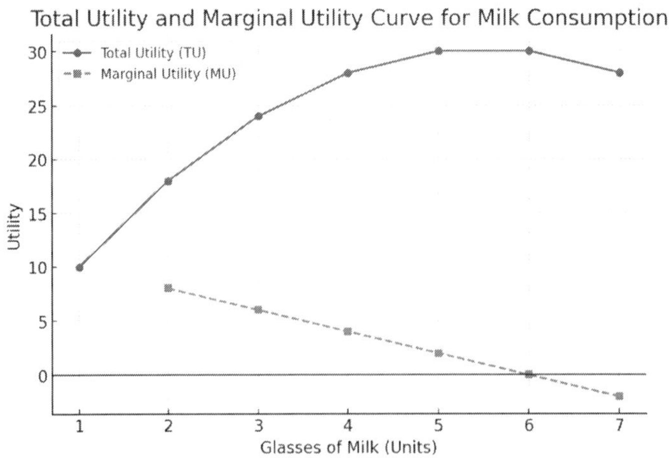

Example in Veterinary Science

1. The first glass of milk is highly satisfying at a given time.
2. The second glass provides some benefit but less than the first.
3. The third glass gives even less benefit, and beyond the fourth or fifth glass, consumption may cause discomfort.
4. Understanding this principle helps in managing livestock feeding and optimizing nutrition for dairy animals.

   This concept is crucial in economic decision-making, consumer behavior analysis, and practical applications such as pricing strategies and dietary planning in animal husbandry.

5. **Practical Applications**

A. Bulk Sales & Discounts

1. The first unit of a commodity (1 glass of milk, dozen eggs, 1kg of meat, or 200 grams of paneer) has high utility.
2. As consumers buy more, additional satisfaction decreases.
3. Businesses offer bulk discounts or loyalty rewards to encourage continued purchases despite diminishing marginal utility.

B. Consumer Equilibrium

1. Consumer equilibrium occurs when a consumer maximizes utility given their budget constraints.
2. When utility is measured in monetary terms, equilibrium is reached when **MU = P** (Marginal Utility equals the Price of the commodity).
3. If **MU > P**, the consumer gains more satisfaction than the price paid, encouraging further consumption.

6. Exceptions to the Law: The Law of Diminishing Marginal Utility may not apply to:
   1. **Precious commodities like gold or money**, where greater quantities increase desirability.
   2. **Experiences such as music or hobbies**, where enjoyment may increase over time.

Summary

Utility is the power of a good or service to satisfy a human want—think of it as the "satisfaction score" you get from consuming something. It's subjective (your score, not mine) and drives why we buy milk or pay a vet. In economics, it's the backbone of consumer behaviour.

Key Point

- Utility = Satisfaction experienced.
- Example: A thirsty farmer consumes an ₹15 water bottle—high utility. A full one skips it—zero utility.

Key Concepts

1. **Total Utility (TU):** Total satisfaction from all units consumed.
   Example: 3 eggs = 30 utils (satisfaction units).
2. **Marginal Utility (MU):** Extra satisfaction from one more unit.
   Example: 1st egg = 15 utils, 2nd = 10, 3rd = 5.
3. **Trends**
   TU rises with more consumption (up to a point).
   MU drops as you add units—enter the Law of Diminishing Marginal Utility.
4. **Law of Diminishing Marginal Utility**
   Definition: This law says: the more you consume of something, the less extra satisfaction each new unit gives—until it hits zero or goes negative. It's why the first bite rocks, but the tenth feels meh.

Core Ideas

1. **Satiability:** One want (e.g., thirst) can be filled—then you're done.
2. **MU Declines:** Extra units lose their magic.
3. **Price Link:** MU reflects what you'd pay—high for the first, less later.

Practical Applications of Law

A. Bulk Sales & Discounts

- **Explanation:** First unit's a thrill—later ones less so. Businesses cut prices to keep you buying.

B. Consumer Equilibrium

- **Explanation:** You max utility when MU = Price—spending matches satisfaction.
  MU > P: Buy more—worth it.
  MU < P: Stop—overpriced.

Assumptions of the Law of Diminishing Marginal Utility

The **Law of Diminishing Marginal Utility** states that as a person consumes more units of a good, the additional satisfaction (marginal utility) derived from each successive unit decreases. This law is based on several key assumptions:

1. **Identical Units of Consumption**

   Each unit of the good consumed should be uniform in quality, size, and nature.

   Example: If a person drinks a glass of milk, the next glass should have the same quantity and taste for the law to hold true because the MU might jump (e.g., if 2nd is creamier).

2. **No Change in Consumer Preferences**

   The consumer's tastes, preferences, and habits should remain constant during the consumption process.

   Example: If a person enjoys eating eggs today but dislikes them tomorrow, the law may not apply correctly.

3. **Continuous Consumption**

   There should be no significant time gap between the consumption of successive units.

   Example: Eating a piece of cheese in the morning and another at night may lead to different hunger levels, altering the satisfaction received.

4. **Standard-Sized Units**

   The units consumed should be of a standard, comparable size.

   Example: Drinking half a glass of milk instead of a full glass may not produce the expected effect on marginal utility.

Exceptions to the Law of Diminishing Marginal Utility

While the **Law of Diminishing Marginal Utility** applies to most goods and services, there are certain exceptions where it does not hold true. Here are some key examples:

1. **Money and Wealth:** Unlike perishable goods, money does not lose its utility as a person accumulates more of it. People's desire for wealth generally increases instead of diminishing.

   Example: A dairy farmer earning ₹ 50,000 per month will still strive to earn more to invest in better cattle, equipment, or land.

2. **Precious Items (Gold, Diamonds):** Luxury items like gold, silver, and diamonds often increase in desirability as people acquire more, mainly due to their status and investment value.

   Example: A farmer who owns one gold ring may still want more jewelry because of its prestige and long-term worth.

3. **Music and Hobbies:** Certain activities, such as music, art, reading, or gardening, may not lose their appeal even after repeated engagement. In fact, enjoyment may increase over time.

   Example: A veterinarian listening to relaxing music while working may appreciate it more over time rather than losing interest.

4. **Addictive Goods (Tea, Coffee, Alcohol, Tobacco):** Addictive substances often defy the law, as repeated consumption increases craving rather than diminishing satisfaction.

Example: A dairy farmer who drinks tea multiple times a day may feel more dependent on it instead of losing interest.

These exceptions illustrate how **utility does not always decrease with additional consumption**, challenging the traditional application of the law in specific cases.

Summary
• **Assumptions:** Same units, steady tastes, no gaps, standard sizes—DMU's foundation. Break them, law falters. • **Exceptions:** Money, gold, hobbies, and addictions— more can mean more utility, not less.

Analytical Questions

1. CASE STUDY: Dairy Farm Expansion and Milk Pricing

Scenario

Rakesh owns a small dairy farm and sells fresh milk to local consumers at ₹50 per liter. Initially, his customers are willing to buy milk at this price. However, as he starts offering bulk discounts for purchases of 5 liters or more, some customers shift to buying in bulk.

Questions

1. *How does the concept of diminishing marginal utility justify Rakesh's decision to offer bulk discounts?*
2. *What pricing strategy should Rakesh adopt to maximize revenue while ensuring that consumers continue purchasing from him?*
3. *If the marginal utility of milk consumption decreases, how can Rakesh add more value to his products to sustain demand?*

Answers

1. The Law of Diminishing Marginal Utility states that as consumers consume more of a product (milk), their additional satisfaction from each extra unit decreases. Offering bulk discounts incentivizes them to buy more despite the declining utility.
2. Rakesh should adopt a tiered pricing strategy—charging ₹50 per liter for small quantities and reducing the price for bulk purchases (e.g., ₹45 per liter for 5 liters or more) to encourage volume sales.
3. To sustain demand, Rakesh can introduce value-added products such as flavored milk, paneer, or ghee, which provide additional utility to consumers beyond just plain milk.

2. CASE STUDY: Poultry Business and Egg Pricing

Scenario

Neha, a poultry entrepreneur, sells eggs at ₹6 per egg. She notices that customers buying in smaller quantities (6 eggs) are willing to pay ₹6 per egg, but those purchasing in bulk (30 eggs) ask for discounts.

Questions

1. *How does the law of diminishing marginal utility explain why bulk buyers demand lower prices?*
2. *If Neha wants to sell more eggs without reducing prices, what strategies can she use?*
3. *If a competitor starts offering eggs at ₹5.50 per egg, how should Neha respond?*

Answers

1. Consumers derive higher satisfaction from the first few eggs they buy. As they buy more, their additional satisfaction per egg decreases, making them less willing to pay the same price per unit. Bulk buyers negotiate lower prices because they value each additional egg less.
2. Neha can bundle eggs with additional benefits such as free home delivery, combo packs (e.g., eggs + poultry feed), or offer loyalty rewards to encourage repeated purchases without reducing prices.
3. Neha can differentiate her eggs by marketing them as organic, free-range, or enriched with Omega-3 to justify her price. Alternatively, she could introduce loyalty programs to retain her customers.

3. CASE STUDY: Veterinary Services and Consumer Behaviour

Scenario

Dr. Amit, a veterinarian, provides consultation services for ₹500 per visit. He notices that pet owners willingly pay for the first consultation but hesitate to return for frequent check-ups at the same rate.

Questions

1. *Why does the demand for frequent consultations decrease according to the Law of Diminishing Marginal Utility?*
2. *How can Dr. Amit encourage pet owners to schedule regular check-ups despite diminishing marginal utility?*
3. *Should Dr. Amit offer a subscription plan for pet health? If so, how should he price it?*

Answers

1. The first consultation provides high utility as it addresses immediate concerns. With repeated visits, the marginal benefit (additional satisfaction) from each consultation decreases unless a new issue arises.
2. Dr. Amit can create value by offering preventive care packages, reminders for vaccinations, and educational sessions on pet health to make regular visits more worthwhile.
3. A subscription plan (e.g., ₹2000 for four visits a year) can encourage customers to commit to regular check-ups while ensuring steady income for the veterinarian.

Exceptions to the Law: Selling Premium Dairy Cows

Question 4

You sell dairy cows at ₹50,000 each, with 5 cows/month demand (MU = 4 utils for 5th cow). Raising to ₹70,000 increases demand to 7 cows as elite farmers seek status. How can you use this exception (Veblen-like) to grow sales?

Answer

Exceptions (e.g., prestige goods) defy diminishing MU—higher prices boost desire.

- **Strategy:** Raise to ₹70,000 and brand as "Elite Herd": "Top cows for top farms." Include a pedigree certificate (₹500 value).
- **Execution:** Market: "₹70,000 = prestige + 20% milk yield—MU rises." Target 5 rich farmers with a seminar (₹5,000 cost), upselling 2 extra cows.
- **Outcome:** Sales hit 10 cows/month (₹7L vs. ₹2.5L), as prestige drives demand up, not down, against the usual MU law.

Bulk Sales & Discounts: Scaling Veterinary Services

Question 5

You offer vet checkups at ₹500/visit, with a farmer's TU peaking at 42 utils for 6 visits (MU = 2 utils). Beyond 6, MU hits 0. How can you apply bulk discounts to overcome diminishing marginal utility and boost bookings?

Answer

Bulk discounts counter MU decline—encourage more purchases.

- **Strategy:** Offer 10 visits at ₹400/visit (₹4,000) with a free vaccine (₹200 value). Pitch: "Full care, lower cost per visit."

- **Execution:** Promote: "6 visits = 42 utils at ₹500; 10 = 45 utils at ₹400—save ₹1,000." Target 5 farmers with a trial (3 visits at ₹450).
- **Outcome:** Bookings rise to 10 visits/farmer (₹4,000 vs. ₹3,000 for 6), up 33%, as discounts offset MU drop.

Total and Marginal Utility: Marketing Egg Packs

Question 6

You sell eggs at ₹6/egg, with a household's TU rising from 15 utils (1 egg) to 30 utils (5 eggs), but MU falls from 15 to 5 utils. They buy 3 eggs/week (MU = 10 utils). How can you use TU and MU to shift them to larger packs?

Answer

TU grows, but MU dims—push bigger packs to max satisfaction.

- **Strategy:** Offer a "Breakfast Pack": 10 eggs at ₹5/egg (₹50). Pitch: "More eggs, more meals—same joy."
- **Execution:** Show value: "3 eggs = 25 utils at ₹18; 10 = 40 utils at₹50—MU drops, but TU soars." Add a free recipe (₹5 value) for 20 buyers.
- **Outcome:** Sales jump to 200 eggs/week (20 x 10 at ₹50 = ₹1,000 vs. ₹360), as higher TU justifies lower MU per egg.

Identical Units of Consumption: Selling Consistent Poultry Feed

Question 7

You sell poultry feed at ₹600/bag, with a farmer's marginal utility (MU) dropping from 12 utils (1st bag) to 4 utils (5th bag) for 5 bags/month. A batch varies in quality, raising MU to 6 utils for the 5th bag. How can you use the identical units assumption to stabilize demand?

Answer

Identical units ensure MU declines predictably—consistency is key.

- **Strategy:** Guarantee uniform quality at ₹600/bag: "Same nutrition, every bag." Offer 6 bags/month at ₹550/bag (₹3,300) with a free scoop (₹50 value).
- **Execution:** Pitch: "5 bags = 40 utils steady—variable quality cheats you." Test with 10 farmers, ensuring each bag matches (e.g., 20% protein).
- **Outcome:** Demand stabilizes at 6 bags/month (₹3,300 vs. ₹3,000), as identical units restore the law's predictable MU drop, boosting trust.

No Change in Preferences: Adapting Dairy Milk Sales

Question 8

You sell milk at ₹60/liter, with a household's MU falling from 15 utils (1st liter) to 5 utils (4th liter) for 4 liters/week. A vegan trend shifts their taste, halting purchases after 2 liters. How can you reinforce steady preferences to maintain demand?

Answer

Stable preferences underpin the law—counter shifting tastes.

- **Strategy:** Keep ₹60/liter and launch "Milk Forever": 5 liters + free recipe book (₹30 value) for ₹300. Pitch: "Stick with dairy—versatile and tasty."
- **Execution:** Promote: "4L = 35 utils if you stay loyal—vegan's a fad." Target 20 households with a tasting event (₹2,000 cost).
- **Outcome:** Demand holds at 100 liters/week (20 x 5L at ₹300 = ₹6,000 vs. ₹4,800), as steady preferences sustain MU decline over units.

Continuous Consumption: Optimizing Veterinary Checkups

Question 9

You offer vet checkups at ₹500/visit, with a farmer's MU dropping from 10 utils (1st visit) to 2 utils (6th visit) weekly. If visits are spaced monthly, MU resets to 8 utils. How can you use continuous consumption to increase bookings?

Answer

Continuous consumption ensures MU dims—tighten visit timing.

- **Strategy:** Offer a "Weekly Health Plan": 8 visits at ₹450/visit (₹3,600/month). Pitch: "Regular care, max value."
- **Execution:** Explain: "6 weekly = 42 utils; monthly resets MU, costs more long-term." Target 5 farmers with a free first visit (₹500 value).
- **Outcome:** Bookings rise to 8 visits/month/farmer (₹3,600 vs. ₹3,000 for 6), as continuous use aligns with the law's MU decline.

Exception - Money and Wealth: Scaling Dairy Investments

Question 10

You sell dairy cows at ₹50,000 each, with a farmer buying 5 cows (MU = 4 utils for 5th). Raising to ₹60,000 increases demand to 6 cows as they see wealth potential. How can you use this money exception to grow sales?

Answer

Money's utility rises with more—leverage wealth desire.

- **Strategy:** Raise to ₹60,000/cow and pitch: "Build wealth—20% milk yield." Offer a "Herd Starter": 8 cows at ₹58,000 each (₹4.64L) with free vet check (₹500 value).
- **Execution:** Market: "More cows, more cash—MU grows." Target 3 rich farmers with a seminar (₹5,000 cost), showing ROI (₹1L/year/cow).
- **Outcome:** Sales hit 8 cows/month (₹4.64L vs. ₹2.5L), as the exception (wealth utility increases) defies diminishing MU.

Exception - Addictive Goods: Marketing Poultry Supplements

Question 11

You sell a poultry vitamin supplement at ₹200/pack, with a farmer's MU dropping from 12 utils (1st pack) to 4 utils (5th pack) for 5 packs/month. After regular use, demand rises to 7 packs at ₹250/pack due to dependency. How can you use this addictive goods exception to boost sales?

Answer

Addictive goods increase utility with use—capitalize on craving.

- **Strategy:** Raise to ₹250/pack and offer a "Flock Boost Plan": 10 packs at ₹230/pack (₹2,300) with free feeder (₹100 value). Pitch: "They'll crave it—lock in gains."
- **Execution:** Promote: "5 packs = 40 utils; 10 = 50 utils—dependency pays." Target 10 farmers with a 5-pack trial (₹1,000).
- **Outcome:** Sales rise to 100 packs/month (10 x 10 at ₹230 = ₹23,000 vs. ₹1,000), as the exception (addictive utility grows) shifts demand up.

Dairy Farm Expansion and Marginal Utility

Ramesh owns a small dairy farm with five cows, producing 50 liters of milk daily. Encouraged by his initial profits, he buys five more cows. However, he notices that the increase in milk production does not proportionally increase his profits due to higher feed costs, labor expenses, and declining market prices.

Question 12

How does the Law of Diminishing Marginal Utility apply to Ramesh's expansion? What factors might be reducing his additional gains?

Answer

The **Law of Diminishing Marginal Utility** applies because each additional cow does not provide the same level of satisfaction or profit as the first few. Factors reducing marginal gains include:

- Increased feeding costs
- Higher labor requirements
- Market saturation leading to lower selling prices
- Limited storage and processing capacity

Ramesh should analyze his input costs and market demand before expanding further.

Poultry Farmer and Egg Production

Scenario

Sita, a poultry farmer, starts with 100 hens, producing 80-90 eggs daily. She notices that as she increases the number of hens to 500, the quality of eggs declines, and disease outbreaks become more frequent, reducing overall profits.

Question 13

Why might Sita be experiencing diminishing marginal utility in her poultry business, and how can she address it?

Answer

The **Law of Diminishing Marginal Utility** explains why increasing production does not always lead to proportional gains. Possible reasons include:

- Overcrowding leading to stress and lower egg quality
- Higher disease susceptibility
- Increased feeding costs without proportionate output

Sita should **invest in better housing, disease management, and nutrition strategies** rather than simply increasing the number of hens.

Veterinary Entrepreneur and Expanding Services

Scenario

Dr. Akash, a veterinary entrepreneur, starts offering consultation services for livestock farmers. Initially, farmers highly value his visits. However, as he increases his workload, he notices that each additional consultation adds less to his income and satisfaction because of longer travel time, fatigue, and reduced personal attention to clients.

Question 14

How does the Law of Diminishing Marginal Utility explain Dr. Akash's situation, and what should he do?

Answer

Dr. Akash is experiencing **DMU because each additional consultation adds less value due to time constraints and fatigue.** To improve efficiency, he should:

- **Introduce digital consultations** to reduce travel time
- **Train assistants** to handle routine cases
- **Prioritize high-value clients** or cases requiring specialized skills

This will allow him to maximize utility from his services rather than overextending himself.

The Exception - Dairy Farmer Investing in Gold

Scenario

Karan, a successful dairy farmer, reinvests his profits in buying gold rather than expanding his farm. Unlike perishable goods, he notices that the value of his gold increases over time.

Question 15

Why does the Law of Diminishing Marginal Utility not apply in Karan's case?

Answer

Gold is an exception to the Law of Diminishing Marginal Utility because:

- It **retains and often increases in value** over time.
- It **acts as a status symbol** and a secure investment.
- Unlike milk or livestock, gold **does not perish or lose appeal** with increased ownership.

Karan's decision is rational for wealth accumulation, but he should ensure diversification in investments.

CASE STUDY: Addiction to Cattle Tonic – An Exception to DMU

Scenario

A group of dairy farmers starts using a special cattle feed supplement that initially improves milk yield. However, over time, the effect diminishes, and they feel compelled to increase the dosage to maintain results.

Question 16

How does this case illustrate an exception to the Law of Diminishing Marginal Utility?

Answer

The case aligns with the **exception of addictive goods**, where repeated use **increases dependence rather than reducing satisfaction.** Farmers may continue using more of the supplement despite declining effects.

To avoid this:

- Farmers should rotate supplements or **consult veterinary nutritionists.**
- Over-reliance on one product **may harm animal health** and **increase costs without proportional benefits.**

6

Theory of Supply & Theory of Costs

Supply is the amount of a good or service sellers are willing to offer for sale at a specific price, in a specific market, over a specific time.

Stock vs. Supply

- **Stock:** All the milk a farmer has—say, 1,000L in tanks.
- **Supply:** What he sells—500L at Rs 50/L today.

Supply is different from stock, as stock refers to the total quantity of a commodity that exists in the market, while supply is the quantity that is usually offered for sale at a particular price.

Law of Supply

The law of supply explains the functional relationship between the price of a good and its supply. When all other factors remain constant, an increase in price leads to an increase in supply. This means there is a direct proportional relationship between price and supply.

Exceptions

1. Land, rare goods, and labour supply in certain cases do not follow the law of supply.
2. The supply of rare goods cannot be changed with price fluctuations.
3. In the case of labour supply, beyond a certain wage level, workers may prefer more leisure instead of working additional hours.

Snippets for better understanding

Supply versus Stock

Supply's about action—what you put out, not what you've got.

Vet Example

- **Stock:** A vet has 100 vaccine doses.
- **Supply:** 20 doses offered at Rs 50 each this week—supply is active, stock is potential.

Law of Supply

The Law of Supply says: *price up, supply up; price down, supply down*—ceteris paribus (all else constant). It's a direct relationship—higher prices tempt producers to sell more.

Why?

- **Profit motive:** Rs 60/L milk beats Rs 50/L—more cows milked, more sold.
- **Positive slope:** Graph it—price (Y-axis) rises, supply (X-axis) follows.

Example:

- **Eggs:** Rs 5/egg = 10,000 eggs supplied/week. Rs 7/egg = 12,000 eggs—farmers ramp up.
- **Vet Fees:** Rs 500/visit = 10 visits/week. Rs 700 = 15 visits—vet works harder.

Change in Supply

There are two types of changes in supply:

1. Extension and contraction of supply
2. Increase and decrease of supply

Extension and Contraction of Supply: When all other factors remain constant, a change in price leads to a change in supply. If the price increases, supply extends. If the price decreases, supply contracts.

Increase and Decrease of Supply: When price remains constant, but other determinants change, supply increases or decreases accordingly.

Determinants of Supply

Supply of a commodity depends on various factors, which are known as determinants of supply:

1. Price of the Goods: The main determinant. Producers supply more goods if prices are high and fewer goods when prices are low.
2. Input Prices: Producers supply more when input prices are low due to lower production costs. Higher input prices lead to lower supply.
3. Technology: Improved technology enhances the supply of goods.
4. Government Policies: Higher taxes discourage production and reduce supply, whereas subsidies encourage producers to increase supply.
5. Expectations about Future Prices: If producers expect future price increases, they may reduce current supply and hoard stock. Conversely, if they anticipate a price drop, they may increase supply.
6. Number of Firms in the Market: Market supply is the sum of the supplies from individual firms. A decrease in the number of firms reduces overall supply.

7. Natural Factors: Supply of goods depends on favorable weather conditions. Droughts, floods, extreme weather, and disease outbreaks can negatively impact supply.

Snippets for Better Understanding

Supply shifts in two ways—price-driven (extension/contraction) or other factors (increase/decrease).

1. **Extension and Contraction of Supply**
   - **Definition:** Price changes, supply adjusts—all else constant.
   - **Extension:** Price rises—supply stretches.
   - **Contraction:** Price falls—supply shrinks.
   - **Vet Example:**
     - **Milk:** Rs 50/L = 500L/day. Rs 60/L = 600L (extension). Rs 40/L = 400L (contraction).
     - **Vet Vaccines:** Rs 50/dose = 20 doses/week. Rs 70 = 30 (extension). Rs 30 = 10 (contraction).
2. **Increase and Decrease of Supply**
   - **Definition:** Price stays put, but other factors shift supply—curve moves right (increase) or left (decrease).
   - **Vet Example:**
     - **Increase:** New milking technology—500L at Rs 50/L jumps to 700L (right shift).
     - **Decrease:** Feed cost spikes—500L at Rs 50/L drops to 300L (left shift).

Graph Peek

- Extension/Contraction: Move *along* the supply curve.
- Increase/Decrease: Shift the *whole curve*.

Key Insight: Price tweaks daily milk sales—tech or costs reshape your whole operation.

Elasticity of supply

Elasticity of supply is the ratio of the proportionate change in the quantity supplied to the proportionate change in price. It measures how responsive supply is to a change in price.

Type of elasticity of supply

1. **Perfectly Elastic Supply:** The quantity supplied changes infinitely with no change in price. Even a slight change in demand can lead to an infinite change in supply, but the price remains constant. Producers are willing to supply any amount of a good or service at a fixed price.

   Example: Suppose the government sets a fixed price for a specific animal vaccine. If demand for the vaccine increases due to an outbreak, manufacturers may supply an unlimited amount at that price.

2. **Relatively Elastic Supply:** The percentage change in quantity supplied is greater than the percentage change in price. A small change in price leads to a larger change in quantity supplied.

   Example: Goods that can be produced quickly or have readily available resources, such as manufactured items, exhibit this. Eggs and chicken have relatively elastic supply. If the price of eggs increases, poultry farmers can quickly increase production by adding more hens or improving feed efficiency.

3. **Relatively Inelastic Supply:** The percentage change in quantity supplied is less than the percentage change in price. A large change in price leads to a smaller change in quantity supplied. This applies to goods that require significant time or resources to produce, such as agricultural products or handmade goods.

   Example: Milk production is relatively inelastic in the short term. Even if the price of milk rises, farmers cannot immediately increase the number of dairy cows or milk production per cow. It takes time to breed more cows or improve herd management.

4. **Unitary Elastic Supply:** The percentage change in quantity supplied is equal to the percentage change in price. The change in supply is proportional to the change in price.

   Example: In some cases, veterinary clinics may adjust their services proportionally to changes in fees. For instance, if the fee for spaying pets increases by 10%, clinics may increase the number of procedures by 10% by hiring additional staff or extending working hours.

5. **Perfectly Inelastic Supply:** The quantity supplied remains constant regardless of changes in price. No matter how much the price changes, the supply does not change. This applies to goods with a fixed quantity, such as original artworks or limited-edition items, where supply cannot increase even if the price rises.

   Example: Certain breeds of cattle or sheep have limited populations. Even if the price of these breeds increases significantly, supply cannot be increased immediately due to the time required for breeding and rearing.

Key Insights in Context

- Perfectly Elastic: Rare in practice but seen in controlled scenarios (e.g., government-fixed prices for dairy or poultry products).
- Relatively Elastic: Common for products with short production cycles (e.g., eggs,).
- Relatively Inelastic: Typical for livestock requiring long rearing times/less shelf life (e.g., milk).
- Unitary Elastic: Occurs when producers can adjust supply proportionally
- Perfectly Inelastic: Applies to fixed or rare resources (e.g., rare breeds, grazing land).

Determinants of Elasticity of Supply

1. Nature of the Commodity

Durable goods (storable) tend to have elastic supply (Es > 1) because producers can stockpile and release them when prices rise. Perishable goods, with short shelf lives, have inelastic supply (Es < 1) due to limited storage potential.

Dairy Example: Cheese vs. Fresh Milk.

Cheese, a durable product, can be stored for months. If cheese prices rise by 10%, dairies can increase supply by 20% by releasing stored stock, making supply elastic. Fresh milk, being perishable, can't be stockpiled long-term—if prices rise, supply barely adjusts (e.g., 5% increase), making it inelastic.

2. Time Factor

Supply is more elastic in the long run (more time to adjust production) and inelastic in the short run (limited adjustment capacity).

Dairy Example: Milk Production

Short term: If milk prices rise by 20%, farmers might only increase supply by 5% by milking cows more frequently—herd size can't grow quickly, so supply is inelastic. Long term: Over years, they can breed more cows, potentially increasing supply by 25%, making it elastic.

3. Availability of Facilities

Good infrastructure (storage, transport, processing) makes supply elastic by enabling quick responses to price changes; poor facilities make it inelastic.

Example: Veterinary Drug Distribution.

In a region with robust supply chains, a 20% price rise for dewormers could increase supply by 30% as distributors ramp up delivery—elastic. In rural areas with poor logistics, supply might rise by 8%, constrained by access, so inelastic.

4. Cost of Production

High production costs reduce elasticity (Es < 1) as suppliers struggle to scale up profitably; low costs increase elasticity (Es > 1).

Dairy Example: Organic Milk vs. Regular Milk.

Organic milk has high costs (certification, premium feed); a 20% price rise might increase supply by 10% due to expense constraints—inelastic. Regular milk, with lower costs, might see a 25% supply jump, making it elastic.

5. Nature of Inputs

Readily available inputs make supply elastic; scarce or specialized inputs make it inelastic.

Poultry Example: Poultry Vaccine Production.

Example: With plentiful raw materials (e.g., antigens), a 20% vaccine price rise could boost supply by 30%—elastic. If inputs are limited (e.g., specialized biologics), supply might rise by 8%, making it inelastic.

6. Risk-Taking

If entrepreneurs are willing to take risks, the elasticity of supply will be higher; otherwise, it will be lower.

Dairy Example: New Dairy Ventures.

Example: If entrepreneurs risk opening new dairies in response to a 20% milk price rise, supply might increase by 30%—elastic. Risk-averse farmers sticking to current herds might only boost supply by 5%, showing inelasticity.

Snippets for Better Understanding

1. **Supply:** What's offered at a price—not total stock.
2. **Law:** Price up, supply up—usually (land, labor can defy).
3. **Changes:** Price shifts = extension/contraction; other factors = increase/decrease.
4. **Determinants:** Price leads—inputs, tech, policy, nature tweak it

Determinants of Elasticity of Supply

1. **Nature of Commodity**: Cheese (elastic) vs. fresh milk (inelastic).
2. **Time Factor**: Long-term egg production (elastic) vs. short-term milk supply (inelastic).
3. **Facilities**: Modern slaughterhouses (elastic) vs. remote vet drug supply (inelastic).
4. **Cost**: Cheap battery eggs (elastic) vs. costly organic milk (inelastic).
5. **Inputs**: Abundant feed (elastic) vs. scarce vaccine materials (inelastic).
6. **Risk**: Bold dairy start-ups (elastic) vs. cautious goat farmers (inelastic).

Theory of cost

Theory of cost: It is the study of the cost function.

Cost Function: The relationship between cost and output is called the **cost function**. For example, in dairy farming, the cost function relates the expenses incurred (feed, labor, veterinary care, etc.) to the output (milk production). In a veterinary clinic, the cost function relates expenses (medical supplies, equipment, labor) to the output (services provided, such as consultations, surgeries, and treatments). Thus in the theory of cost, we relate costs to units of output.

Cost

1. Cost refers to the total amount of funds used in production. The cost of production arises because the supply of productive resources is scarce relative to their demand.

For example, in any production process—like raising livestock or running a veterinary clinic—resources such land, building, water, labour, and equipment are limited (scarce). Because these resources are in demand by many producers (farmers, vets, etc.), they come with a cost.

2. The cost of production is always related to a specific time period (e.g., monthly feed expenses, annual salaries).
3. Costs in any production period include the value of resource services transferred into the product during that single period, rather than the value of the resources themselves. This means the cost isn't about what the resources are worth on their own (e.g., the price tag of a tractor or a bag of feed), but what their services contribute to the final product—like healthy animals, eggs, or milk—during a set time. It's about the *use* of the resource, not its total value.For example: A ₹5-lakh tractor's cost is not recorded as ₹5 lakh in one year—instead, its depreciation (e.g., ₹50,000/year) is the cost.
4. Mono-period resources: These are resources which are entirely transformed into the product (or completely used up) in a single production period. For example in dairy farming concentrate feed and fodder are mono-period resources
5. For mono-period resources, their entire value constitutes the cost of production. . In a vet clinic, medical supplies costs vaccines, bandages, and medications used up in a single period. For example, if a clinic spends Rs 1 lakh on vaccines in a year, this is the cost.
6. Poly-period resources are resources whose productive services can be used over many periods.
7. For poly-period resources only the portion used in a single production period constitutes the cost of production. For example in a vet clinic equipment like X-ray machines and surgical tools are used over many years. If an X-ray machine costs 30,0000 and lasts10 years, the annual cost is Rs 30,000/-

Importance of Cost Concepts

1. The cost of production also provides guidance in setting adequate and remunerative prices. For example a dairy farmer calculates the total cost of milk production (feed, labor, veterinary care, etc.) to set a profitable selling price per liter of milk. If production cost is ₹40 per liter, pricing must be above this to ensure profitability.

2. For efficient resource use, a farm needs to select the least-cost combination of resources for each level of output. Cost concepts are essential for determining the least-cost, optimal combination of resource use.

   Let's say you need to vaccinate 100 cows against a disease. You have two options:

   i. Option A: Buy a bulk vaccine for Rs 500 and hire an assistant for Rs 200 to help administer it. Total cost = Rs 700.

   ii. Option B: Buy individual doses for Rs 800 and do it yourself (no extra labor cost). Total cost = Rs 800.

   iii. Both options achieve the same output (100 vaccinated cows), but Option A's cost is lower (Rs 700 vs. Rs 800). By analyzing costs, you pick the least-cost combination—bulk vaccine plus an assistant—for efficient resource use.

3. The quantity of a product that a farm will supply to the market depends on the cost of production. The lower the per-unit cost of production, the greater the incentive for producers to increase supply. Imagine you offer a Artificial Insemination service. Initially, your cost per cow is Rs 100 (Straw cost + travel + time), and you charge Rs 150, making Rs 50 profit per cow. You inseminate 20 cows monthly, supplying 20 AI services. Then, you find a cheaper straw supplier and transport cost, dropping your cost to Rs 75 per cow. Now, your profit per cow is 75 per cow. This lower per-unit cost motivates you to expand—maybe hiring help to inseminate 50 cows monthly—because the incentive (higher profit) is greater.

The term "cost" isn't just one thing—it varies depending on what you're measuring: cash spent, sacrifices made, or even societal impacts. For veterinarian and farmers, understanding these helps you manage money, make smart decisions, and see the bigger picture of production.

Key Takeaways

- **Cost Function:** Ties cash spent (feed, tools) to output (milk, vet services).
- **Cost:** Scarcity's price—monoperiod (feed Rs 1,000) used up, polyperiod (cattle shed Rs 50,000/year) spread out.

Importance: Sets prices, picks efficiency, drives supply (lower cost = more milk).

1. Money cost

Definition: This is the actual cash you spend on production—real money transactions to pay for resources like labour, feed, or equipment.

Example: A dairy farmer pays:

- Rs 10,000/month as wages to workers milking cows.
- Rs 5,000/month for cattle feed.
- Total money cost = Rs 15,000/month.

These are tangible expenses you see in your bank account—straightforward and tied to physical payments.

Application: If you're a vet running a clinic, money costs include Rs 2,000 for vaccines and Rs 3,000 for a receptionist's salary. Tracking these helps you set service fees.

2. Real costs

This isn't about money but the sacrifices, effort, or hardships involved in production. It's the "pain" or trade-offs you endure. It considers the **human effort** required in running an enterprise.

Example: For a dairy farmer:

- Long hours spent milking cows instead of resting.
- Physical strain from lifting heavy feed bags.
- Emotional stress if a cow falls sick.

Thus, a dairy farmer waking up early, working long hours, and facing physical fatigue in managing cattle are real costs.

Application: A vet student might face real costs like sleepless nights studying for exams or the effort of traveling to remote farms for fieldwork. It's not cash, but it's a real burden.

3. Economic cost

It is the total cost of production, which includes.

I. Explicit cost – Direct cash payments (like money cost).

II. Implicit cost- The values of resources owned by producer (self-owned land, personal capital).

III. Normal profit- The minimum profit required to keep a business running.

Example: A dairy farmer:

- **Explicit Cost:** A farmer **buys feed** for Rs 8,000/month.
- **Implicit Cost:** Uses his own land (worth Rs 5,000/month if rented out) instead of leasing it.
- **Normal Profit:** Expects Rs 10,000/month to justify staying in dairy farming.

- Economic Cost=Explicit Cost+ Implicit Cost+ Normal Profit
- **Economic Cost:** Rs 8,000 + Rs 5,000 + Rs 10,000 = Rs 23,000/month.

Application: A vet using her own car (worth Rs 2,000/month rental value) for farm visits has an implicit cost, plus explicit costs like Rs 1,000 for gas, and needs Rs 5,000 profit to keep going. Economic cost = Rs 8,000/month.

Types of Implicit Costs

Implicit costs often involve what you give up by choosing one option over another. Two key types:

a) Opportunity cost

The value of the next best alternative you forgo when you make a choice.

Example 1: A farmer with 5 acres of land can:

- Grow fodder for cattle (50 tons/year).
- Or grow wheat (20 quintals/year).
- If he picks fodder, the opportunity cost is 20 quintals of wheat he didn't produce.

Example 2: A farmer with Rs 1 lakh can:

- Invest in a dairy farm (earns Rs 15,000/year).
- Or start a poultry farm (earns Rs 20,000/year).
- Choosing dairy means an opportunity cost of Rs 20,000 (poultry profit lost).

b) Depreciation

Definition: The loss in value of your own equipment or assets over time due to use.

Example: A vet buys a Rs 50,000 ultrasound machine that lasts 5 years. Each year, it depreciates by Rs 10,000. That's an implicit cost if she owns it, not a cash payment.

Applications of opportunity cost

1. **Determination of Factor Prices:** Workers, land, or capital must earn at least what they could in their next best use, or they'll shift elsewhere.

   Example: A dairy farmer pays workers Rs 10,000/month. If a nearby poultry farm offers Rs 12,000, workers might leave unless the dairy farmer matches that opportunity cost (Rs 12,000). The entrepreneur must **match or exceed** this wage to retain workers.

2. **Determination of economic rent:** The **difference between actual earnings and opportunity cost** of a factor. The extra income a resource earns above its opportunity cost.

   Example: A farmer uses crossbreed cows (10 liters milk/day) instead of indigenous cows (5 liters/day). If crossbreeds earn Rs 5,000/month more, that's economic rent—extra profit beyond the indigenous option's value.

3. **Consumer decision making:** Given a fixed income, consumers must decide how to allocate spending among different goods. Consumers weigh trade-offs with limited money.

Example: A buyer with Rs 100 can buy fresh cow milk (Rs 50/liter) or packaged milk (Rs 40/liter). Choosing fresh milk means the opportunity cost is the packaged milk (and Rs 10 left unspent).

4. Private cost & social cost

Private cost: Costs borne by the producer—direct expenses for running the operation.

Example: A poultry farmer's private costs:

- Feed: Rs 5,000/month.
- Wages: Rs 3,000/month.
- Vaccines: Rs 1,000/month.
- Total: Rs 9,000/month.

Social cost: The total cost to society, including external effects like pollution or health risks.

Example

A poultry farm buys feed, pages ways and mange vaccination costs- These are private cost.

If farm improperly dispose of poultry waste, leading to water pollution, it imposes a social cost on the nearly community.

If social cost is higher than private cost, regulations may be needed to ensure environmental and public health protection. A vet clinic using loud equipment might annoy neighbours (a social cost), even if the clinic's private costs (electricity, tools) are low. Regulations might step in to balance this.

Recap of Key Terms

i. **Explicit Costs:** Cash payments (e.g., Rs 8,000 for feed). Also called accounting or cash costs.

ii. **Implicit Costs:** Value of your own resources (e.g., Rs 5,000 for using your land). Non-cash costs.

iii. **Normal Profit:** The minimum profit to stay in business (e.g., Rs 10,000/ month).

i.	**Money Cost:** Cash you pay—Rs 15,000 for feed and wages.
ii.	**Real Cost:** Sweat and stress—late nights milking cows.
iii.	**Economic Cost:** Full price tag—Rs 23,000 (cash + own land + must-have profit).
iv.	**Explicit Cost:** Money out—Rs 8,000 for vet supplies.
v.	**Implicit Cost:** Hidden sacrifices—Rs 5,000 land value you don't rent out.
vi.	**Opportunity Cost:** What you skip—Rs 20,000 poultry profit lost for dairy.
vii.	**Depreciation:** Wear and tear—Rs 10,000/year off your tractor.
viii.	**Normal Profit:** Bare minimum—Rs 10,000 to keep farming.
ix.	**Private Cost:** Your tab—Rs 9,000 for poultry feed and labor.
x.	**Social Cost:** Society's bill—Rs 11,000 with pollution added.

Time element and cost

The time element plays a crucial role in the analysis of production costs and supply in economics. The classification of time periods into *very short-period, short period, and long period* helps in understanding how firms adjust their production levels and costs in response to changes in demand.

Very Short-Period (Market Period)

i. **Definition**: This is the shortest period during which firms **cannot change output** levels. The supply is fixed and limited to **existing stock**.

ii. **Adjustment**: No inputs can be changed.

iii. **Price Determination**: Prices are determined solely by **demand**.

Example: Fresh milk in the market today — supply can't be increased quickly.

3. Short Period

i. **Definition**: A period where firms can **adjust only variable inputs** like labour and raw materials, but **not fixed inputs** like buildings or machinery.

ii. **Output Adjustment**: Possible, but constrained.

iii. **Costs**: Both fixed and variable.

4. Long Period

i. **Definition**: Sufficient time for firms to **change all inputs**, including fixed ones. They can **scale operations up or down**.

ii. **Adjustment**: Full flexibility.

iii. **Technology and Infrastructure**: Can be updated or replaced.

Relationship between Time Periods and Costs

Relationship between Time Periods and Costs

Time Period	Cost Characteristics
Very Short-Period	Costs are largely **fixed**.
Short Period	Costs are **fixed + variable**.
Long Period	**All costs become variable** and adjustable.

Long Period Costs

I. Total Fixed Costs

i. **Definition**: Total Fixed Costs (TFC) are expenses that **do not change** with the level of output (production). These costs must be paid **even if output is zero** because they are associated with **fixed inputs** (e.g., land, machinery, salaries).

ii. **Other Names:** Indirect costs, Supplementary costs, sunk costs (if already incurred and non-recoverable),overhead costs (general business expenses not tied to production volume)

iii. **Examples**: Expenditure on land, buildings, salaries of permanent employees, interest payments, and insurance premiums.

iv. **Implication**: Fixed costs are unavoidable and must be covered even if the firm produces nothing.

Example

Units of Output (Milk production in litres)	Total Fixed Costs
0	50,000
100	50,000
200	50,000
300	50,000
400	50,000
500	50,000

Total Fixed Cost Curve: A horizontal line parallel to the x-axis, indicating that fixed costs remain constant at all levels of output.

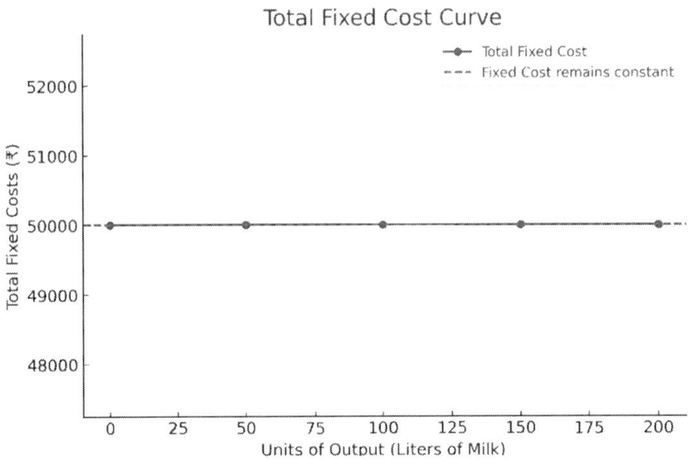

II. Total Variable Costs (TVC)

1. **Definition**: Total Variable Costs (TVC) are expenses that change directly with the level of output (production). These costs increase when output rises and decrease when output falls. If production stops (zero output), TVC becomes zero.
2. **Key Characteristics:** Directly linked to production volume (more output = higher variable costs).Can be adjusted in the short run (unlike fixed costs).
3. **Examples:** costs of raw materials, wages for temporary labour, maintenance charges of machinery, electricity, fuel, and veterinary medicines.
4. Also known as working costs, operating costs, direct costs, prime costs, circulating costs and running costs
5. **Implications**

   Zero when production is zero (no feed used if no chicken is produced, no medicines used if no animals are treated).

   Higher production = higher variable costs (but efficiency can reduce per-unit costs initially).

   Critical for profit calculation (Revenue – (Fixed Costs + Variable Costs) = Profit).

Example Table (Poultry Farm)

Number of Chickens Raised	Total Variable Costs (₹)
0	0
100	5,000
200	9,500
300	15,000

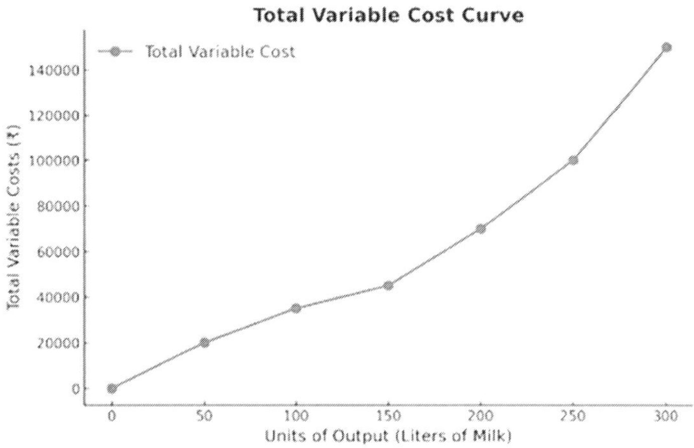

Total Variable Cost Curve (TVC Curve)

i. **It starts from the origin (0, 0)** → No output means no variable costs.

ii. **Initially concave (increasing at a decreasing rate)** → Due to **economies of scale** (e.g., bulk feed discounts, efficient labour use).

iii. **Later becomes convex (increasing at an increasing rate)** → Due to **diminishing returns** (e.g., overcrowded poultry farms needing more medicine, overtime labour costs).

iv. **Graphically it is inverse "S" shaped curve**

III. Total Costs (TC)

Total Cost (TC) is the *sum of all expenses* incurred in production. It includes the two components of total fixed cost and total variable cost

i. **Total Fixed Costs (TFC)** → Do not change with output (e.g., rent, salaries).

ii. **Total Variable Costs (TVC)** → Change with output (e.g., feed, medicines).

Formula: TC=TFC+TVC

i. Total cost and rate of increase of total cost is same as that of total variable cost as one of the two components (i.e. total variable cost) remains constant

ii. The rate of increase in TC is the same as that of TVC because TFC remains constant.

iii. The Total Cost Curve and the Total Variable Cost Curve have similar shapes.

iv. The only difference is that:

a) The TVC curve starts from the origin (0, 0).

b) The TC curve starts from a positive intercept, which equals the Total Fixed Cost.

c) Initially, the TC curve is concave, and later, it becomes convex due to the law of variable proportions.

Example Table (Dairy Farm):

Litres of Milk Produced	TFC (₹)	TVC (₹)	TC (₹) = TFC + TVC
0	50,000	0	50,000
100	50,000	20,000	70,000
200	50,000	35,000	85,000
300	50,000	55,000	105,000

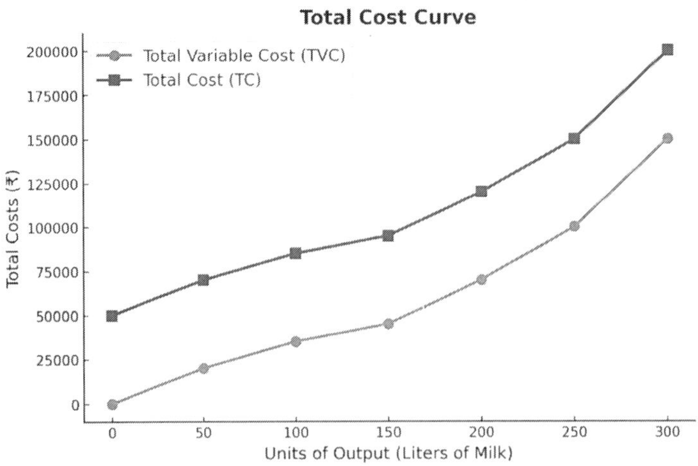

IV. Average Fixed Cost (AFC)

1. **Definition**: It is total fixed cost divided by the quantity of output. It can also be said to be the cost of fixed resources or inputs required for producing one unit of output.

   a) AFC=Total Fixed Costs/ Output S

2. **Average Fixed cost curves**

   i. Since total fixed cost remains same as output rises, average fixed cost diminishes but never becomes zero.

   ii. As output approaches zero ,the average fixed cost curve approaches infinity so curve never touches either of the axis

   iii. **AFC Curve**: A downward-sloping curve that approaches the x-axis but never touches it.

   iv. **Mathematically, AFC is a rectangular hyperbola** → Approaches both axes asymptotically.

Example Table (Poultry Farm)

Chickens Produced (Q)	TFC (₹)	AFC (₹) = TFC/Q
100	1,00,000	1,000
1,000	1,00,000	100
5,000	1,00,000	20
10,000	1,00,000	10

V. Average Variable Cost (AVC)

1. Definition: It is the total variable cost divided by the quantity of output.

   a) AVC=TVC/Output

2. Average output rises, the **AVC Curve** first falls, reaches a minimum and then begins to rise. So AVC curve has a U shape.

Units of Production	TVC (₹)	AVC
100	1,00,000	1,000
1,000	1,00,000	100
5,000	1,00,000	20
10,000	1,00,000	10

VI. Average Total Cost (ATC)

1. **Definition**: Total cost divided by the quantity of output. It is the sum of AFC and AVC.

   a) ATC=TC/Output=AFC+AVC

2. ATC decreases initially due to falling AFC and AVC but eventually increases due to rising AVC.
3. **ATC Curve**: U-shaped, similar to the AVC curve but lies above it due to the inclusion of AFC.

VII. Marginal Cost (MC)

- **Definition**: The change in total cost due to a one-unit change in output.

  MC=ΔTCΔ/Output

Behaviour

Marginal cost curve is also U shaped. This is explained by law of variable proportion which says that with increase in a variable factor, keeping other factors constant, marginal physical product first increases and then after a certain level of production, it starts to decline.Initially decreases due to increasing returns to scale but eventually increases due to diminishing returns.

- **MC Curve**: U-shaped, intersecting the AVC and ATC curves at their minimum points.

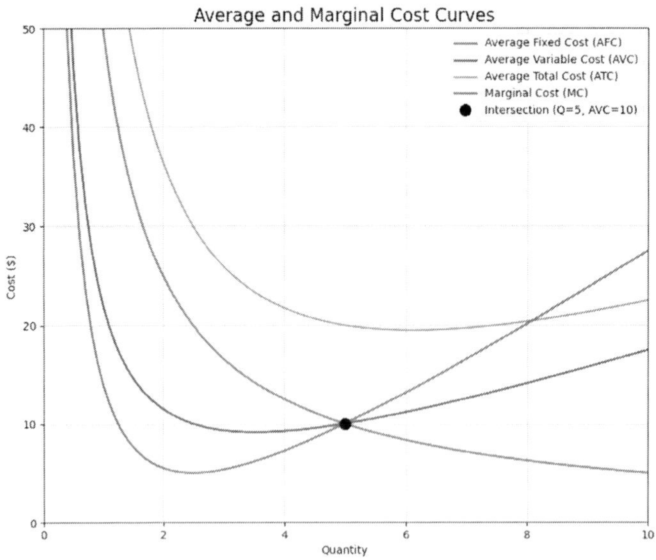

Various Types of Costs: Key Takeaways

1. Total Fixed Cost: They're tied to fixed inputs—like land or machinery—and you pay them even if output is zero. Think of them as the "base rent" of production.
2. Total Variable Cost (TVC): TVC flexes with your dairy herd—zero output, zero cost; scale up, it climbs.
3. Total cost: Total Cost is the full tab—TFC + TVC. It's all expenses, fixed and variable, to produce your output.
   TC curve rises with TVC (since TFC's flat)—same pace, different starting point.
4. Average Fixed Cost: Average fixed cost is TFC spread over output—cost per unit for fixed inputs.
5. Average Variable Cost is TVC per unit of output.
   - **Formula:** AVC = TVC ÷ Output
   - **Key Feature:** U-shaped—falls, hits a low, then rises.
6. Average Total Cost is TC per unit—combines AFC and AVC.
   - **Formula:** ATC = TC ÷ Output = AFC + AVC
   - **Key Feature:** U-shaped—falls early (AFC drop), rises later (AVC climb).
7. Marginal Cost is the extra cost of one more unit of output.
   - **Formula:** MC = ΔTC ÷ Δ Output
   - **Key Feature:** U-shaped—law of variable proportions drives it.
   - **TFC:** Fixed Rs 50,000—flat line.
   - **TVC:** Scales with output—0 to Rs 15,000, S-shaped.
   - **TC:** TFC + TVC—Rs 50,000 start, climbs with TVC.
   - **AFC:** Falls forever—Rs 1,000 to Rs 10.
   - **AVC/ATC:** U-shaped—find the dip.
   - **MC:** U-shaped—guides extra output.

Summary of Cost Concepts

Cost Type	Definition	Behaviour	Curve Shape
Fixed Costs (FC)	Costs that do not vary with output.	Constant at all levels of output.	Horizontal line parallel to x-axis.
Variable Costs (VC)	Costs that vary with output.	Increase as output increases; zero when output is zero.	Upward-sloping curve.
Total Costs (TC)	Sum of fixed and variable costs.	Increase as output increases.	Upward-sloping curve starting from TFC.
Average Fixed Cost (AFC)	TFC divided by output.	Decreases as output increases.	Downward-sloping curve.
Average Variable Cost (AVC)	TVC divided by output.	Initially decreases, then increases.	U-shaped curve.
Average Total Cost (ATC)	TC divided by output.	Initially decreases, then increases.	U-shaped curve.
Marginal Cost (MC)	Change in TC due to a one-unit change in output.	Initially decreases, then increases.	U-shaped curve intersecting AVC and ATC at their minimum points.

Analytical Questions

Question 1

Suggest few examples of fixed costs in a veterinary clinic, poultry farm and dairy farm?

Industry	Fixed Cost Examples
Veterinary Clinic	Rent of clinic, salaries of permanent staff, medical equipment loans, insurance, licensing fees.
Poultry Farm	Poultry shed depreciation, loan payments on land, salaries of farm managers, biosecurity system costs.
Dairy Farm	Milking machine costs, barn construction expenses, veterinary service contracts, property taxes

Question 2

Suggest few examples of variable costs in a veterinary clinic, poultry farm and dairy farm?

Industry	Variable Cost Examples
Veterinary Clinic	Medicines, disposable syringes, lab tests, temporary staff wages.
Poultry Farm	Poultry feed, vaccines, day-old chicks, electricity for heating, casual labor.
Dairy Farm	Cattle feed, milking supplies, veterinary medicines, artificial insemination costs.

Question 3

Why understanding various costs concept matters for Vet and Animal Husbandry Students

i. Money Cost: Helps you budget and track cash flow—vital for a clinic or farm.

ii. Real Cost: Reminds you of the personal effort behind the job.

iii. Economic Cost: Shows the full picture, including hidden costs, to set fair prices or decide if a venture's worth it.

iv. Opportunity Cost: Guides choices—like whether to raise goats or sheep, or invest in a vet degree vs. a farm.

v. Private vs. Social Cost: Highlights your responsibility to the community (e.g., managing waste or noise).

Question 4

Discuss a CASE STUDY: How a Vet Clinic Used Cost Analysis to Double Profits?

Background

GreenPaws Veterinary Clinic (Small Animal Practice)

- **Location:** Semi-urban area
- **Services:** Consultations, surgeries, vaccinations, grooming
- **Problem:** Struggling with **low profits** despite high patient flow.

Step 1: Analysing Money Costs (Explicit Costs)

The clinic tracked **all cash expenses** for 3 months:

Cost Category	Monthly Expense (₹)
Rent	25,000
Salaries (2 vets + 1 assistant)	80,000
Medicines & Supplies	60,000
Equipment Maintenance	10,000
Utilities (Electricity/Water)	8,000
Total Money Cost	1,83,000

Finding

- Clinic needed **₹1.83L/month** just to break even.
- Revenue averaged **₹2.2L/month** → Profit = **₹37,000 (only 17% margin)**.

Step 2: Identifying Hidden Costs (Implicit + Opportunity Costs)

1. **Implicit Cost**
   - Owner (Head Vet) didn't pay herself a salary.
   - **Opportunity Cost:** She could earn **₹50,000/month** working at a corporate clinic.
2. **Depreciation**
   - Ultrasound machine (₹5L) depreciated by **₹5,000/month**.
3. **Normal Profit**
   - Owner expected **at least ₹40,000/month** to justify running the clinic.

Revised Economic Cost

₹1,83,000 (Money Cost)+₹50,000 (Opportunity Cost)+₹5,000 (Depreciation)+₹40,000 (Normal Profit) =**₹2,78,000/ month**₹1,83,000

(Money Cost)+₹50,000 (Opportunity Cost)+₹5,000 (Depreciation) +₹40,000 (Normal Profit)=**₹2,78,000/*month***

The clinic was **losing ₹58,000/month** economically.

Step 3: Cost-Cutting & Efficiency Strategies

A) Reduce Money Costs

1. **Negotiated with Suppliers**
    - Switched to generic medicines → Saved **₹15,000/month**.
2. **Cross-Trained Staff**
    - Assistant learned basic grooming → Reduced outsourcing costs by **₹8,000/month**.
3. **Energy Efficiency**
    - Installed solar panels → Cut electricity bills by **₹3,000/month**.

B) Optimize Opportunity Costs

- **Added Teleconsultations**
- Used idle time for online consults → Earned extra **₹20,000/month**.
- **Sublet Unused Space**
- Rented out a room to a pet food seller → **₹10,000/month**.

C) Price Adjustments

- **Value-Based Pricing**
- Charged **20% more for emergency services** (demand was inelastic).
- Introduced **preventive care packages** (e.g., ₹5K/year for vaccinations + checkups).

Results after 6 Months

Metric	Before	After
Monthly Revenue	₹2,20,000	₹3,50,000
Monthly Money Costs	₹1,83,000	₹1,45,000
Gross Profit	₹37,000	₹2,05,000
Economic Profit	-₹58,000	+₹67,000

Key Improvements

1. **Profit Doubled:** From ₹37K to ₹2.05L (gross).
2. **Economic Profit Achieved:** Now earning **₹67K** above opportunity cost.
3. **Sustainable Model:** Preventive care packages ensured steady cash flow.

Lessons

Track All Costs: Hidden costs (like your unpaid labor) can make a profitable business seem unviable.

1. **Cut Waste:** Small savings (like switching to generics) add up.
2. **Diversify Revenue:** Teleconsults, subletting, and packages optimize resource use.
3. **Price Smartly:** Charge based on value, not just cost.

5. Question

A dairy farm experiences a sudden increase in demand for milk due to a festival. Explain how the farm can respond in the very short-period, short period, and long period. What are the constraints in each period?

Answer

Very Short-Period

i. The farm cannot increase milk production immediately because the number of cows and their milk yield are fixed.

ii. The supply is limited to the existing stock of milk.

iii. **Constraint**: Fixed & variable factors like, number of sheds, the number of cows and milking equipment cannot be changed.

Short Period

i. The farm can increase milk production by improving the feed of cows, hiring additional labour for milking, fodder harvesting.

ii. Constraint: Fixed factors like barn size and milking machinery cannot be changed.

Long Period

i. The farm can expand its operations by purchasing more cows, building additional barns, or investing in advanced milking technology.

ii. Constraint: No constraints; all factors of production can be adjusted.

6. Question

A poultry farm faces a surge in demand for eggs during winter. Analyze how the farm can adjust its production in the short period and long period. What are the key differences in cost structure between these two periods?

Answer

Short Period

i. The farm can increase egg production by adding more lighting to stimulate egg-laying, improving feed quality, or hiring temporary workers.

ii. **Cost Structure**: Variable costs (feed, labor, electricity) increase, but fixed costs (coops, machinery) remain unchanged.

Long Period

i. The farm can expand its operations by building new coops, purchasing more chickens, or investing in automated feeding systems.

ii. **Cost Structure**: All costs become variable, including the cost of new infrastructure and equipment.

- **Key Difference**: In the short period, only variable costs can be adjusted, while in the long period, both variable and fixed costs can be changed.

7. Question

A pet clinic experiences a sudden increase in patients due to an outbreak of a contagious disease. How can the clinic manage this situation in the very short-period, short period, and long period? What are the challenges in each period?

Answer

Very Short-Period

- The clinic cannot immediately expand its capacity. It can only serve patients based on existing resources (veterinarians and examination rooms).
- **Challenge**: Limited by fixed factors like the number of veterinarians and clinic space.

Short Period

- The clinic can extend working hours, hire part-time staff, or optimize the use of existing resources.
- **Challenge**: Fixed factors like clinic size and full-time staff cannot be changed.

Long Period

- The clinic can expand by building new examination rooms, hiring more full-time veterinarians, or investing in advanced medical equipment.
- **Challenge**: Requires significant investment and planning.

Question 8

A feed manufacturing company faces a sudden increase in demand for animal feed due to a disease outbreak in poultry. How can the company adjust its production in the short period and long period? What are the implications for its cost structure?

Answer

Short Period

- The company can increase production by running extra shifts, hiring temporary workers, or optimizing raw material usage.
- **Implications**: Variable costs (labor, raw materials) increase, but fixed costs (factory rent, machinery) remain unchanged.

Long Period

- The company can expand its operations by building a new factory, purchasing advanced machinery, or sourcing more raw materials.
- Implications: All costs become variable, including the cost of new infrastructure and equipment.

Question 9

A veterinary pharmaceutical company experiences a sudden increase in demand for a specific drug due to an outbreak of a disease in livestock. Analyze how the company can respond in the very short-period, short period, and long period. What are the limitations in each period?

Answer

Very Short-Period

- The company cannot increase production immediately. It can only supply the existing stock of the drug.
- **Limitation**: Fixed factors like production capacity and raw material availability cannot be changed.

Short Period

- The company can increase production by running extra shifts, hiring temporary workers, or optimizing raw material usage.
- **Limitation**: Fixed factors like factory size and machinery cannot be changed.

Long Period

- The company can expand its operations by building a new production facility, investing in advanced manufacturing technology, or sourcing more raw materials.
- **Limitation**: Requires significant investment and time.

Question 10

Why is the distinction between fixed costs and variable costs important for businesses in the dairy, poultry, and pharmaceutical industries? Provide examples from each industry to support your answer.

Answer

Importance

- Fixed costs (e.g., machinery, buildings) remain constant regardless of production levels, while variable costs (e.g., labor, raw materials) change with production. Understanding this distinction helps businesses plan production, manage costs, and make decisions about scaling operations.
- **Examples**
- **Dairy Industry**: Fixed costs include barns and milking equipment; variable costs include feed and labor.
- **Poultry Industry**: Fixed costs include coops and machinery; variable costs include feed and electricity.
- **Pharmaceutical Industry**: Fixed costs include factory rent and equipment; variable costs include raw materials and labor.

Sunita runs a small dairy farm . She keeps detailed records of her monthly costs: ₹25,000 on feed, ₹10,000 on labor, ₹5,000 on veterinary care, and ₹10,000 on utilities and depreciation. Her 10 cows produce 3,000 liters of milk per month.

Question 11

How can Sunita derive her cost function, and how should it guide her milk pricing?

Answer

- **Total Cost** = ₹25,000 (feed) + ₹10,000 (labor) + ₹5,000 (vet) + ₹10,000 (others) = ₹50,000
- **Output** = 3,000 liters
- **Cost per liter** = ₹50,000 / 3,000 = ₹16.67

Cost function (simplified)

C(Q) = 16.67Q, where Q = liters of milk

To make a profit, she must **price her milk above ₹16.67/liter**, considering demand and competition.

CASE STUDY 1 Mono-Period and Poly-Period Resources in a Veterinary Clinic

Scenario

Dr. Meena runs a rural veterinary clinic. In one year, she uses:

- **₹1,20,000 on vaccines and medicines**
- **₹30,000 on bandages and syringes**
- **She also uses a ₹3,00,000 ultrasound machine with a useful life of 10 years.**

Question 12

Identify mono-period and poly-period resources and calculate annual cost.

Answer

Mono-period resources (used up in a year):

- Medicines & vaccines = ₹1,20,000
- Bandages/syringes = ₹30,000
- Total mono-period cost = ₹1,50,000

Poly-period resource (used over years):

- Ultrasound machine = ₹3,00,000/10 = ₹30,000 per year

Annual total cost = ₹1,50,000 + ₹30,000 = ₹1,80,000

This cost helps her decide pricing for consultations, surgeries, and treatment services.

CASE STUDY 2: Choosing the Least-Cost Combination in Poultry

Scenario

Amit wants to expand his poultry farm's vaccination coverage for 1,000 birds.

- **Option A: Bulk vaccine = ₹3,000 + labor ₹1,000 = ₹4,000**
- **Option B: Small-dose vaccine packs = ₹4,500 (no labor cost)**

Question 13

Which option should he choose, and why?

Answer

- **Option A cost per bird** = ₹4,000 / 1,000 = ₹4
- **Option B cost per bird** = ₹4,500 / 1,000 = ₹4.5

Option A is more economical. The principle of least-cost combination favors this choice as both options yield the same output (1,000 vaccinated birds) but A has a lower cost.

CASE STUDY 3: Cost Influencing Supply in AI Services

Scenario

Dr. Raj performs Artificial Insemination (AI) services at ₹150 per cow. His earlier cost was ₹100 per cow (Rs 50 profit). By shifting to a local semen supplier and carpooling, he reduces his cost to ₹75.

Question 14

What impact does this cost reduction have on his business decisions?

Answer

- **Profit rises from ₹50 to ₹75 per cow.**
- Increased profit **motivates him to expand** services from 20 to 50 cows per month.

This shows that **a fall in per-unit cost increases supply** and encourages scaling up.

CASE STUDY 4: Understanding Depreciation in a Dairy Farm

Scenario

Manoj purchases a milking machine for ₹2,00,000 with a life of 10 years. He also spends ₹1,20,000 yearly on feed and ₹30,000 on labor.

Question 15

What is the annual cost of the machine and how is it recorded?

Answer

- The machine is a **poly-period resource**.
- **Annual depreciation** = ₹2,00,000 / 10 = ₹20,000
- It is this **₹20,000 (not ₹2,00,000)** that is included in the **annual cost of production.**

This prevents overestimating cost in a single year and aligns cost with service usage.

CASE STUDY 5: Pricing Based on Production Cost

Scenario

Nisha produces 2,000 eggs/month at a cost of ₹6 per egg. The market price is ₹5.50 per egg.

Question 16

Should she continue production at this cost?

Answer

No. Her **cost per unit (₹6)** is **higher than the selling price (₹5.50)**, leading to a **loss of ₹1,000/month**. She should:

- Cut costs (e.g., cheaper feed, bulk purchase)
- Increase efficiency
- Consider value-addition (e.g., selling boiled eggs, tray packing)

CASE STUDY 6: Opportunity Cost in Veterinary Services

Scenario

Dr. Anita can either spend Sunday doing mobile vet services (earning ₹5,000) or attend a local seminar to improve her skills.

Question 17

What is the opportunity cost of attending the seminar?

Answer

The **opportunity cost** is **₹5,000**, which she **sacrifices** by choosing professional development over income. While not a direct cost, it's crucial in decision-making.

CASE STUDY 7: Societal Cost in Poultry Waste Disposal

Scenario

A poultry entrepreneur disposes of farm waste near a village stream, causing water pollution.

Question 18

What kind of cost is this and why should it be considered?

Answer

This is a **social cost**—a **negative externality** not reflected in the entrepreneur's private expenses. It may result in:

- Public health issues
- Legal actions
- Loss of reputation

Responsible waste disposal should be included in cost planning to avoid future liabilities.

CASE STUDY 8: Dairy Farm Cost Planning

Scenario

Rohit owns a small dairy farm with 6 cows. Every month, he incurs the following:

- **Feed cost: ₹6,000**
- **Labor wages: ₹8,000**
- **Electricity and water bills: ₹1,000**
- **He uses his own land, which he could have rented for ₹4,000/month.**
- **He expects a normal profit of ₹6,000/month to continue in business.**

Question 19

What is Rohit's money cost? What is his implicit cost? What is his economic cost?

Answer

- Money Cost = ₹6,000 (feed) + ₹8,000 (labor) + ₹1,000 (utilities) = ₹15,000
- Implicit Cost = ₹4,000 (rental value of own land)
- Economic Cost = Explicit Cost + Implicit Cost + Normal Profit = ₹15,000 + ₹4,000 + ₹6,000 = ₹25,000/month

CASE STUDY 9: Real Cost in Veterinary Practice

Scenario

Dr. Meena, a rural veterinary officer, travels 20 km daily to remote areas to treat livestock. She receives a salary, but:

- **She works 10–12 hours a day.**
- **She faces poor road conditions.**
- **She misses family time and suffers from fatigue.**

Question 20

What type of cost is Dr. Meena facing beyond her salary? Why is this cost important to consider when evaluating her contribution?

Answer

- **Real Cost** – This includes the physical, emotional, and mental sacrifices (long hours, fatigue, travel).
- It's important because **real costs reflect non-monetary inputs** and help in **evaluating job satisfaction and policy support needed** for rural vets.

CASE STUDY 10: Opportunity Cost in Poultry Farming

Scenario

Priya owns 3 acres of land. She can either:

- **Use the land to grow maize for her poultry (worth ₹20,000/year), or**
- **Lease it for wheat cultivation (rent income ₹30,000/year).**

Question 21

If she chooses to grow maize, what is her opportunity cost?If maize contributes more to her poultry business than ₹30,000/year, is it a wise decision?

Answer

- **Opportunity Cost = ₹30,000 (forgone rental income from wheat farming)**
- Yes, if maize as poultry feed contributes more than ₹30,000 in profits/ savings, it is a wise decision.

CASE STUDY 11: Depreciation in a Vet Clinic

Scenario

A vet clinic buys a surgical laser machine for ₹2,00,000. The expected life is 10 years.

Question 22

What is the annual depreciation cost? Is this depreciation an implicit or explicit cost?

Answer

- **Depreciation = ₹2,00,000 ÷ 10 = ₹20,000/year**
- Since the machine is owned and not rented, depreciation is an **implicit cost**.

CASE STUDY 12: Private and Social Costs in Poultry Farming

Scenario

A commercial poultry farm spends:

- **₹10,000 on feed**
- **₹4,000 on labor**
- **₹1,000 on vaccines**

However, it disposes of waste in a nearby water stream, causing foul smell and contamination.

Question 23

What is the private cost? Identify a social cost involved. What should the entrepreneur do to reduce social costs?

Answer

- Private Cost = ₹10,000 (feed) + ₹4,000 (labor) + ₹1,000 (vaccines) = ₹15,000
- Social Cost = Water pollution, foul smell, health hazard to nearby villagers
- The entrepreneur should **invest in proper waste management** (e.g., composting or biogas unit) to reduce external harm and **avoid penalties or community backlash**.

CASE STUDY 13: Price Setting Based on Economic Cost

Scenario

A dairy entrepreneur calculates the following monthly costs:

- **Feed: ₹9,000**
- **Labor: ₹6,000**
- **Own land (could rent for ₹5,000)**
- **Normal profit expectation: ₹10,000**
- **Monthly milk output: 1,000 liters**

Question 24

What is the per-liter cost of milk production using the economic cost method?

Answer

- **Total Economic Cost = ₹9,000 + ₹6,000 + ₹5,000 (implicit) +₹10,000 (normal profit) = ₹30,000**

- **Per-liter cost = ₹30,000 ÷ 1,000 liters = ₹30/liter** To make profit, the selling price must be **above ₹30/liter**.

CASE STUDY 14: Choosing Between Dairy & Poultry Enterprise

Scenario

- **Rajan has ₹2 lakhs to invest.**
- **Dairy Option: ₹25,000/year return**
- **Poultry Option: ₹40,000/year return**

He chooses dairy because it's his passion.

Question 25

What is the opportunity cost of his decision?What is his implicit cost?

Answer

- Opportunity Cost = ₹40,000 – ₹25,000 = ₹15,000/year (forgone poultry profit)
- Implicit cost includes not just monetary sacrifice, but emotional and time investments in dairy that could have been spent elsewhere.

CASE STUDY 15 Money Cost: Setting Veterinary Service Fees

Question 26

You run a vet clinic with monthly money costs of ₹15,000 (₹10,000 staff wages, ₹5,000 medical supplies). You serve 50 clients/month at ₹400/visit, but rising supply costs push expenses to ₹18,000. How can you use money cost to adjust pricing and maintain profitability?

Answer

Money cost reflects cash outlays—price above it for profit.

- **Strategy:** New per-visit cost: ₹18,000 ÷ 50 = ₹360. Raise fees to ₹450/visit (₹90 profit/visit). Pitch: "Top care, fair price."
- **Execution:** Break down costs: "₹360 covers supplies and staff—₹450 ensures quality." Offer a 5-visit pack at ₹425/visit (₹2,125) to lock in 10 clients.
- **Outcome:** Revenue rises to ₹22,500/month (50 x ₹450) vs. ₹20,000, profit to ₹4,500 vs. ₹5,000, covering money cost increase while staying competitive.

CASE STUDY 16: Real Cost: Balancing Dairy Farming Efforts

Question 27

You're a dairy farmer spending ₹20,000/month on feed and labor (money cost) for 1,000 liters of milk, sold at ₹50/liter. Real costs include 12-hour days and physical strain, causing burnout. How can you address real costs to sustain operations?

Answer

Real costs are sacrifices—reduce effort without raising money cost.

- **Strategy:** Keep ₹20,000 budget but hire a part-time worker (₹5,000/month) to cut hours from 12 to 8/day. Maintain ₹50/liter price.
- **Execution:** Reallocate: ₹15,000 feed, ₹5,000 labor. Pitch: "Same fresh milk, rested farmer." Train worker to handle milking (₹1,000 one-time cost).
- **Outcome:** Output holds at 1,000 liters (₹50,000 revenue), profit ₹30,000, while real cost (strain) drops, ensuring long-term viability.

CASE STUDY 17: Economic Cost: Scaling Poultry Egg Production

Question 28

You produce 2,000 eggs/month with explicit costs of ₹8,000 (feed ₹6,000, wages ₹2,000) and sell at ₹6/egg. Implicit costs include your land (₹3,000/month rental value) and normal profit expectation (₹5,000). Demand rises to 3,000 eggs. How can you use economic cost to set a sustainable expansion plan?

Answer

Economic cost (explicit + implicit + normal profit) guides total pricing needs.

- **Strategy:** Current economic cost: ₹8,000 + ₹3,000 + ₹5,000 = ₹16,000 (₹8/egg). For 3,000 eggs: explicit ₹12,000, implicit ₹3,000, profit ₹5,000 =₹20,000 (₹6.67/egg). Sell at ₹7/egg.
- **Execution:** Pitch: "₹7/egg—fresh, farm-direct." Boost feed (₹9,000), wages (₹3,000) efficiently. Market to 10 new buyers.
- **Outcome:** Revenue ₹21,000 (3,000 x ₹7), economic cost ₹20,000, profit ₹1,000 above normal, ensuring expansion covers all costs.

CASE STUDY 18. Opportunity Cost: Choosing Between Dairy and Poultry Ventures

Question 29

You have ₹1 lakh to invest. Dairy farming yields ₹15,000/year profit (10 cows), while poultry offers ₹20,000/year (1,000 chicks). You choose dairy, but costs rise, cutting profit to ₹12,000. How can you use opportunity cost to reassess and optimize your decision?

Answer

Opportunity cost is the forgone alternative—re-evaluate based on returns.

- **Strategy:** Opportunity cost of dairy = ₹20,000 (poultry profit). Switch to poultry: ₹20,000/year vs. ₹12,000. Start with 500 chicks (₹50,000) + ₹50,000 savings. Sell eggs at ₹6 (₹10,000/year profit).
- **Execution:** Pitch: "Eggs beat milk—higher returns." Liquidate 5 cows (₹25,000), fund chicks. Test with 10 farmers buying 100 eggs/month.
- **Outcome:** Profit rises to ₹10,000/year (500 eggs/month x ₹6 - ₹20,000 cost), beating dairy's ₹12,000, aligning with opportunity cost logic.

CASE STUDY 19: Private Cost vs. Social Cost: Managing Poultry Waste

Question 30

Your poultry farm produces 1,000 kg of meat/month with private costs of ₹30,000 (feed ₹20,000, labor ₹10,000), sold at ₹200/kg. Improper waste disposal pollutes a local river, adding ₹5,000/month in social costs (cleanup). How can you address private and social costs to sustain operations?

Answer

Private costs are yours; social costs hit society—balance both for viability.

- **Strategy:** Keep ₹ 200/kg but invest ₹2,000/month in a waste composter, reducing social cost to ₹1,000 (monitoring). Total private cost:₹ 32,000.
- **Execution:** Pitch: "Clean farm, quality meat—₹200/kg." Compost waste into fertilizer (₹1,000 revenue/month). Educate locals (₹500 cost) to avoid regulations.
- **Outcome:** Revenue ₹2,00,000, private cost ₹32,000, profit ₹1,68,000, social cost minimized to ₹1,000, ensuring sustainability and community goodwill.

CASE STUDY 20. Very Short-Period: Managing Milk Stock during a Festival

Question 31

You're a dairy farmer with 500 liters of milk in stock (TFC = ₹20,000) during a festival week (very short-period). Demand spikes to 700 liters, but you can't increase output. How can you use the very short-period concept to maximize revenue?

Answer

In the very short-period, supply is fixed—adjust pricing to demand.

- **Strategy:** Raise price from ₹50/liter to ₹ 70/liter due to fixed 500L stock. Pitch: "Festival special—limited stock."
- **Execution:** Promote: "500L only—₹70/L for fresh milk." Target bulk buyers (e.g., sweet shops) with 50L orders at ₹65/L (10 orders). Costs: TFC ₹20,000 (no TVC, stock-based).
- **Outcome:** Revenue hits ₹35,000 (500 x ₹70) vs. ₹25,000, profit ₹ 15,000 vs. ₹5,000, as fixed supply leverages high demand.

CASE STUDY 21. Short Period: Scaling Poultry Feed Production

Question 32

You produce 1,000 kg of poultry feed/month (TFC = ₹50,000, TVC = ₹30,000, TC = ₹80,000) sold at ₹100/kg. Demand rises to 1,200 kg, but your factory (fixed) limits expansion. How can you use short-period costs to meet demand profitably?

Answer

In the short period, vary variable inputs (TVC) within fixed capacity.

- **Strategy:** Increase TVC to ₹36,000 (extra labor ₹4,000, raw materials ₹2,000) for 1,200 kg. Keep ₹100/kg. TC = ₹86,000. Pitch: "More feed, same quality."
- **Execution:** Hire temp workers (₹4,000), bulk-buy materials (₹2,000 savings). Promote: "1,200 kg ready—₹100/kg." AVC = ₹30/kg (₹36,000 ÷ 1,200).
- **Outcome:** Revenue ₹1,20,000 (1,200 x ₹100), profit ₹34,000 vs. ₹20,000, as short-period TVC adjustment meets demand.

CASE STUDY 22. Long Period: Expanding Veterinary Clinic Capacity

Question 33

You run a vet clinic with TFC = ₹1,00,000 (rent, equipment), TVC = ₹50,000 (supplies, staff), serving 200 clients/month at ₹1,000/visit. Demand grows to 300 clients, and all factors can vary. How can you use long-period costs to scale efficiently?

Answer

In the long period, all costs are variable—optimize scale.

- **Strategy:** Expand: new equipment (TFC to ₹1,50,000), staff/supplies (TVC to ₹75,000), TC = ₹2,25,000 for 300 clients. Keep ₹1,000/visit. ATC = ₹750/client.
- **Execution:** Pitch: "More slots, same care—₹1,000/visit." Lease bigger space (₹50,000/year), hire vet (₹25,000). Market to 50 new farmers.
- **Outcome:** Revenue ₹3,00,000 (300 x ₹1,000), profit ₹75,000 vs. ₹50,000, as long-period flexibility lowers ATC and boosts capacity.

CASE STUDY 23: Average Fixed Cost (AFC) and Average Variable Cost (AVC): Pricing Dairy Products

Question 34

You produce 200 liters of milk/month (TFC = ₹40,000, TVC = ₹20,000, TC = ₹60,000), sold at ₹350/liter. Output rises to 400 liters (TVC = ₹36,000, TC = ₹76,000). How can you use AFC and AVC to adjust pricing competitively?

Answer

AFC falls, AVC varies—price to cover costs and compete.

- **Strategy:** For 400L: AFC = ₹100/L (₹40,000 ÷ 400), AVC = ₹90/L (₹36,000 ÷ 400), ATC = ₹190/L. Lower price to ₹250/L (₹60/L profit). Pitch: "More milk, better deal."
- **Execution:** Promote: "₹250/L—fresher, cheaper." Bulk discount: 50L at ₹240/L for 5 buyers. Spread TFC over higher output.
- **Outcome:** Revenue ₹1,00,000 (400x ₹250), profit ₹24,000 vs. ₹10,000 (200 x ₹350 - ₹60,000), as falling AFC and stable AVC support lower pricing.

CASE STUDY 24: Marginal Cost (MC): Optimizing Poultry Egg Supply

Question 35

You produce 2,000 eggs/month (TC = ₹10,000, TFC = ₹4,000, TVC = ₹6,000) sold at ₹6/egg. Adding 500 eggs raises TC to ₹11,000 (MC = ₹2/

egg). Demand hits 3,000 eggs. How can you use MC to increase supply profitably?

Answer

MC reflects cost per extra unit—supply more if MC < price.

- **Strategy:** Produce 3,000 eggs: TC = ₹12,000 (TFC ₹4,000, TVC ₹8,000), MC = ₹2/egg (₹2,000 ÷ 1,000 extra eggs). Keep ₹6/egg. ATC = ₹4/egg. Pitch: "More eggs, same price."
- **Execution:** Add feed (₹1,500), labor (₹500). Promote: "₹6/egg—stock up." Target 10 new buyers with 50-egg packs. MC < ₹6 = profit incentive.
- **Outcome:** Revenue ₹18,000 (3,000 x ₹6), profit ₹6,000 vs.₹2,000, as low MC drives higher supply and profit.

CASE STUDY 25: Dairy Entrepreneur – Time Element and Cost Management

Case: Ramesh runs a small dairy unit in Himachal Pradesh with five cows. Recently, he observed an increase in the demand for milk during the local festival season. However, he could not increase milk production immediately.

Question 36

Identify the time period (very short, short, or long) applicable in Ramesh's situation and explain why he couldn't meet the rise in demand.

Answer

Ramesh is in the **Very Short-Period (Market Period)**. During this period, supply cannot be increased because production levels are fixed. He cannot instantly increase the number of lactating cows or their milk yield, hence he is constrained by the existing stock.

CASE STUDY 26: Poultry Farm – Fixed and Variable Costs

Case: Shalini runs a poultry farm with 1,000 birds. She pays ₹1,00,000 as rent and salaries (fixed costs), and spends ₹1,00,000 on feed, medicines, and power (variable costs). She plans to raise production by increasing the number of birds to 2,000.

Question 37

Differentiate between her fixed and variable costs and explain what changes as she increases her production.

Answer

- **Fixed Costs:** ₹1,00,000 for rent and permanent staff (do not change with output).
- **Variable Costs:** ₹1,00,000 for feed, medicines, etc. (change with output). When she increases her birds to 2,000, **variable costs will increase** (more feed, medicine, etc.), but **fixed costs will remain the same** unless she expands infrastructure.

CASE STUDY 27: Veterinary Entrepreneur – Marginal Cost Decisions

Case: Dr. Arjun provides mobile veterinary services. He currently serves 20 villages at a total cost of ₹40,000. Serving one more village increases his cost to ₹42,000.

Question 38

Calculate the Marginal Cost (MC) of serving the additional village. Should Dr. Arjun consider expansion if his additional revenue per village is ₹2,500?

Answer

- MC = Change in Total Cost / Change in Output = (₹42,000 – ₹40,000) / 1 = ₹2,000
- Since **MC (₹2,000) < Additional Revenue (₹2,500)**, Dr. Arjun should **expand**, as it adds to profit.

CASE STUDY 28: Cost Curve Understanding for a New Dairy Unit

Case: A new dairy entrepreneur in Kangra produces 0, 100, 200, and 300 litres of milk per day. His fixed cost is ₹50,000. His total variable cost is ₹0, ₹20,000, ₹35,000, and ₹55,000 respectively.

Question 39

Construct a Total Cost (TC) table and explain the shape of the Total Cost Curve

Answer

Output (litres)	TFC (₹)	TVC (₹)	TC = TFC + TVC (₹)
0	50,000	0	50,000
100	50,000	20,000	70,000
200	50,000	35,000	85,000
300	50,000	55,000	105,000

Total Cost Curve starts from ₹50,000 (fixed cost) and rises with output.

- It is initially **concave**, then **convex**, due to increasing then diminishing returns.

CASE STUDY 29: Understanding Average Costs in Poultry

Case: Priya raises 1,000 chickens. Her fixed cost is ₹1,00,000. Her variable cost is also ₹1,00,000. She expands her farm to raise 5,000 chickens, keeping fixed cost the same.

Question 40

Calculate AFC, AVC, and ATC at 1,000 and 5,000 chickens. Comment on efficiency.

Answer

Chickens	TFC	TVC	AFC (TFC/Q)	AVC (TVC/Q)	ATC (AFC+AVC)
1,000	₹1,00,000	₹1,00,000	₹100	₹100	₹200
5,000	₹1,00,000	₹1,00,000	₹20	₹20	₹40

Efficiency Increases: As output increases, all average costs decrease, showing economies of scale.

CASE STUDY 30: Veterinary Product Business – Law of Variable Proportion

Case: A veterinary medicine supplier increases his sales agents from 5 to 10, then 15, keeping office and warehouse fixed. Sales initially increase rapidly, then stagnate due to overcrowding and duplication of work.

Question 41

Which economic law explains this, and how does it affect cost curves?

Answer

This is explained by the **Law of Variable Proportions**. Initially, more variable inputs (agents) lead to **increasing returns**, lowering average costs. Beyond a point, **diminishing returns** set in, increasing **marginal cost (MC)** and **average costs**.

CASE STUDY 31: Long Run Decision – Dairy Infrastructure Expansion

Case: Sohan has run a small dairy unit for three years and is considering building a larger shed and purchasing automated milking machines to increase production from 200 to 500 litres/day.

Question 42

Which time period is relevant here? How will this affect the cost structure?

Answer

This is a **Long Period** decision. All inputs can be varied. Fixed costs will rise (new shed, machinery), but over time, **average total costs may decrease** due to **economies of scale** and improved efficiency.

CASE STUDY 32: Decision on Optimum Output – Dairy Processing Unit

Case: Kiran owns a small dairy that also produces paneer. Her cost data shows:

- **Producing 50 kg paneer costs ₹10,000**
- **Producing 100 kg paneer costs ₹17,000**
- **Producing 150 kg paneer costs ₹27,000**

Her revenue from selling paneer is ₹ 200/kg.

Question 43

At what output level should Kiran produce to maximize profit? Show marginal cost and marginal revenue.

Answer

Output	Total Cost	Marginal Cost	Revenue	Marginal Revenue
50 kg	₹10,000	–	₹10,000	–
100 kg	₹17,000	₹7,000	₹20,000	₹10,000
150 kg	₹27,000	₹10,000	₹30,000	₹10,000

- At **100 kg**, MR > MC ⇒ Expand
- At **150 kg**, MR = MC ⇒ **Profit-maximizing output**

Kiran should produce **150 kg paneer** to maximize profits.

CASE STUDY 33: Cost of Delay – Veterinary Consultant

Case: Dr. Preeti provides AI (artificial insemination) services in remote villages. She delays her visits by a week due to roadblocks. Farmers miss timely heat detection, leading to 20 missed AI opportunities.

Question 44

Which type of cost does this represent, and how can it be minimized?

Answer

This is an example of **Opportunity Cost** — the **loss of income or benefit due to delay**.

- Missed income = 20 x ₹300 (AI charges) = ₹6,000
- Can be minimized by **using local para-vets**, teleconsultation, or alternate transport plans.

CASE STUDY 34: Poultry – Economies of Scale

Case: Ravi owns a broiler farm of 2,000 birds. He plans to expand to 6,000 birds and invest in a semi-automatic feeder and waterer. His friend warns him about diseconomies at scale.

Question 45

Explain the concepts of economies and diseconomies of scale in Ravi's case

Answer

- **Economies of Scale**: Per bird cost reduces due to bulk buying, automation, shared fixed costs.
- **Diseconomies of Scale**: May arise if labor is inefficient, disease spreads faster, or supervision becomes poor.

Ravi should expand **gradually**, ensuring **biosecurity** and **trained labor** to retain economies of scale.

CASE STUDY 35: Cost Curve Interpretation – Dairy

Case: Geeta runs a mini dairy. She finds that increasing milk production from 100 to 200 litres/day decreases her average cost from ₹50/litre to ₹35/litre. Beyond 300 litres, cost rises to ₹42/litre.

Question 46

Sketch and interpret her Average Cost Curve. What should be her optimum scale of operation?

Answer

- **U-shaped Average Cost Curve**: First falls due to increasing returns, then rises due to diminishing returns.
- Optimum scale = **Output at minimum point of AC curve** = **Around 200-300 litres/day**

Geeta should maintain production at this level for maximum cost efficiency.

CASE STUDY 36: Shutdown Decision – Poultry Hatchery

Case: A small hatchery faces low demand for chicks during monsoon. Per month:

- **Fixed Cost = ₹1,50,000**
- **Variable Cost = ₹1,00,000**
- **Revenue = ₹2,00,000**

Question 47

Should the hatchery shut down temporarily or continue operations?

Answer

- Total Cost = ₹2,50,000
- Revenue = ₹2,00,000 ⇒ **Loss = ₹50,000**

But revenue **covers variable costs and part of fixed costs**. Hence, **continue operations** in short run to reduce fixed cost burden.

CASE STUDY 37: Break-even Point for Goat Dairy

Case: A goat entrepreneur sells milk at ₹60/litre. Fixed cost/month = ₹30,000. Variable cost/litre = ₹30.

Question 48

Calculate Break-Even Output in litres.

Answer

Break-even Output = Fixed Cost / (Selling Price – Variable Cost)

= ₹30,000 / (₹60 – ₹30)

= **1,000 litres**

The entrepreneur must sell **1,000 litres/month** to break even.

CASE STUDY 38: Long-Term Expansion – Veterinary Diagnostic Lab

Case: Dr. Nisha wants to open a regional veterinary diagnostic lab. It requires land, equipment, staff, and regulatory clearances.

Question 49

Explain the cost and time period considerations for such a project

Answer

- This is a **Long Period** decision: All inputs (land, capital, labor) are variable.
- High **initial fixed costs**, but per test cost can reduce with volume (economies of scale).
- Need proper **break-even and ROI analysis** before investment.

CASE STUDY 39: Sunk Cost – Failed Feed Mill Project

Case: A poultry feed entrepreneur invested ₹10 lakhs in setting up a plant. Due to faulty equipment, it failed. He considers whether to reinvest or start afresh.

Question 50

Should the initial investment affect his future decision? What is a sunk cost?

Answer

- ₹10 lakh is a **Sunk Cost** – **irrecoverable past expense**.
- Decision should be based on **future returns**, not past losses.
- He should ignore the sunk cost and **evaluate fresh feasibility**.

Types of Elasticity of Supply in Dairy, Poultry, and Animal Husbandry

Question 51

What is perfectly elastic supply, and how might it apply to my dairy business?

Answer

Perfectly elastic supply means you can supply an infinite amount at a fixed price, but any price drop stops supply entirely. For a dairy entrepreneur, this could apply to **government-subsidized bulk milk powder**. If the government sets a fixed price (e.g., \$0.30/kg) and demand spikes due to an export deal, you could process and supply unlimited milk powder from surplus milk at that price. But if the price falls below \$0.30, production stops as it's unprofitable—supply is perfectly elastic at that fixed point.

Question 52

How does relatively elastic supply work for a poultry entrepreneur?

Answer

Relatively elastic supply means a small price increase leads to a larger supply increase (elasticity > 1). For your poultry business, consider **egg production**. If egg prices rise by 15% (e.g., from \$2 to \$2.30 per dozen), you could boost supply by 25% by adding hens or improving feed efficiency within weeks. The short production cycle makes your egg supply relatively elastic, letting you capitalize on price hikes quickly.

Question 53

As a veterinary entrepreneur, what's an example of relatively inelastic supply in my field?

Answer

Relatively inelastic supply means a large price increase results in a small supply increase (elasticity < 1). For you, **milk production support services** (e.g., lactation consulting for dairy farms) might fit. If your fees rise by 20% due to demand, you can't instantly increase services by much—say, only 5%—because training more staff or expanding your herd coverage takes time, making supply relatively inelastic in the short term.

Question 54

How does unitary elastic supply apply to my dairy processing venture?

Answer

Unitary elastic supply means the percentage change in supply matches the price change (elasticity = 1). In your dairy business, **cheese production** could be an example. If cheese prices rise by 10% (e.g., from $5 to $5.50/kg), you might increase supply by 10% by reallocating milk from yogurt to cheese production. This proportional adjustment reflects unitary elasticity, balancing your response to market shifts.

Question 55

What's perfectly inelastic supply, and how might it affect my poultry breeding business?

Answer

Perfectly inelastic supply means supply stays fixed no matter the price change (elasticity = 0). For your poultry business, **heritage turkey breeds** are a case. If turkey prices jump by 40% before Thanksgiving, you can't increase supply beyond your current flock—say, 500 birds—because breeding more takes months or years. This fixed supply limits your ability to profit from price surges.

Determinants of Elasticity of Supply in Dairy, Poultry, and Veterinary/ Animal Husbandry

Question 56

How does the nature of the commodity affect my dairy supply decisions as an entrepreneur?

Answer

Durable goods have elastic supply, while perishables are inelastic. If you deal in **cheese** (durable), a 10% price rise could let you increase supply by 20% by releasing stored stock—elastic supply helps you profit. But with **fresh milk** (perishable), the same price rise might only boost supply by 5% since you can't store it long—its inelasticity limits quick gains, pushing you to focus on steady sales.

Question 57

As a poultry entrepreneur, how does the time factor influence my supply elasticity?

Answer

Supply is inelastic short-term but elastic long-term. If **chicken meat** prices rise by 25%, you might only increase supply by 10% in 6–8 weeks (broiler growth time)—inelastic due to time constraints. Over a year, you could expand your flock and boost supply by 30%, making it elastic. Plan short-term efficiency tweaks and long-term growth to match market trends.

Question 58

How do facilities impact my veterinary supply business elasticity?

Answer

Good facilities make supply elastic; poor ones keep it inelastic. If you run a **veterinary drug distribution** business with cold storage and fast transport, a 20% price rise for vaccines could increase supply by 30%—elastic due to infrastructure. In a rural area with no storage, supply might rise by 8%, staying inelastic. Invest in logistics to boost responsiveness.

Question 59

Why does cost of production matter for my organic dairy startup's supply elasticity?

Answer

High costs make supply inelastic; low costs make it elastic. For your **organic milk**, high feed and certification costs mean a 20% price rise might only increase supply by 10%—inelastic due to expense barriers. Compare this to regular milk, where lower costs could let you raise supply by 25%. To grow, focus on cost efficiencies or niche premiums.

Question 60

How does the nature of inputs affect my poultry feed production as an entrepreneur?

Answer

Available inputs increase elasticity; scarce ones reduce it. If **corn and soy** for your feed are plentiful, a 15% price rise could boost supply by 22%—elastic thanks to easy sourcing. If a drought limits supply, the same price rise might only increase output by 6%—inelastic. Secure reliable input suppliers to keep your supply flexible.

Question 61: ***As a veterinary clinic owner, how does risk-taking influence my service supply elasticity?***

Answer

Risk-taking boosts elasticity; caution limits it. If you're willing to open a new clinic in a rural area after a 20% fee increase, you could raise service supply by 35%—elastic due to bold expansion. If you avoid the risk fearing low demand, supply might grow by 10% (e.g., extra hours at your current site)—inelastic. Weigh risks vs. market potential to scale effectively.

Question 62: ***How do these determinants combine for my dairy-poultry hybrid business?***

Answer

Imagine you produce **butter** (dairy) and **eggs** (poultry). Butter's durability and good facilities might make supply elastic (e.g., 15% price rise, 25% supply increase), but high organic feed costs could limit egg supply elasticity (e.g., 15% price rise, 8% supply increase). Short-term, both are inelastic due to time; long-term, both can grow elastic with investment. Balance facility upgrades and cost management to optimize both.

7

Theories of Production

Production- Function- The technical law relating inputs to outputs has been given the name of production function. Production function expresses the relationship between physical input and physical output of a firm for a given state of technology.

Law of Variable Proportion or Law of Diminishing Returns (Short Run Production Function)

This law explains the relationship between inputs and outputs in the short period. According to this law, output can be changed by altering variable factors (such as labour and feed) while keeping other factors (such as land and infrastructure) constant. The law states that with an increase in variable factors, keeping other factors constant, total product initially increases at an increasing rate, then increases at a diminishing rate, and finally starts decreasing.

1. **Total Product (TP)** - Refers to the total output of the firm per period of time.
    1. Example: Total litres of milk produced by a dairy farm per day.
2. **Average Product (AP)** - It is the total output per unit of the variable input. AP is calculated as:

    AP = TP/L (Where TP = Total Product, L = Labor)

    1. Example: If a farm produces 100 liters of milk with 5 cows, AP = 100/5 = 20 liters per cow.
3. **Marginal Product (MP)** - It is the change in the total product resulting from using an additional unit of the variable factor.

    MP = d(TP)/dL (Rate of change of TP with respect to labour)

    1. Example: If adding one extra worker increases daily milk production from 100 litres to 110 litres, MP = 10 litres.

Explanation of the Law with Example

When one factor (e.g., labour, feed) increases while others remain constant (e.g., barn size, equipment), production follows three stages:

Stage 1: Increasing Returns

1. Total Product increases at an increasing rate due to better utilization of resources.
2. Marginal Product increases because more labour improves efficiency.
    1. **Example:** Adding more workers to a dairy farm improves milking efficiency, leading to higher milk yield per cow.

Stage 2: Diminishing Returns (Optimal Stage)

1. TP continues to increase but at a decreasing rate.
2. MP starts to decline but remains positive.
    1. **Example:** Increasing the feed quantity beyond a certain point still increases milk production, but the rate of increase slows down as cows reach their maximum digestive capacity.

Stage 3: Negative Returns

1. TP starts declining as MP becomes negative.
2. Overcrowding or excessive feeding leads to stress, inefficiency, or wastage, causing lower overall production.
    1. **Example:** If too many cows are placed in a limited shed, stress and competition reduce milk yield.

Diagrammatic Explanation

1. **Stage I** – TP increases at an increasing rate, MP is rising.
2. **Stage II** – TP increases at a decreasing rate, MP starts to decline.
3. **Stage III** – TP declines, MP becomes negative.

Key Observations

1. In the first stage, TP, AP, and MP increase, but at the end of the stage, MP starts to decline. This stage ends when MP equals AP.
2. In the second stage, TP increases at a diminishing rate, AP decreases, and MP declines. At the end of this stage, TP reaches its maximum, and MP becomes zero (intersects the x-axis).
3. In the third stage, TP and AP decline, while MP becomes negative and crosses the x-axis.
4. The MP curve intersects the AP curve when AP is at its maximum.

The **Law of Variable Proportions** suggests that optimal resource allocation is critical. Farmers and entrepreneurs should operate in **Stage 2 (Diminishing Returns)** where output is maximized before inefficiencies set in. Excessive use of variable inputs (like labor, feed, or space) beyond a point leads to inefficiencies and even reduces output.

Explanation of Law of Variable proportion through Table & Graph

Consider a **fixed factor** (Land = 1 acre) and a **variable factor** (Labour). The table below shows how Total Physical Product (TPP) and Marginal Physical Product (MPP) change as more units of labour are added.

Fixed Factor (Land in Acres)	Variable Factor (Labour in Units)	Total Physical Product (TPP)	Marginal Physical Product (MPP)	Stage
1	0	0	-	-
1	1	2	2	Stage I
1	2	6	4	Stage I
1	3	12	6	Stage I
1	4	16	4	Stage II
1	5	18	2	Stage II
1	6	18	0	Stage II
1	7	14	-4	Stage III
1	8	8	-6	Stage III

Law of Returns to Scale

This is an important concept that explains how output changes when all inputs (factors of production) are increased proportionally in the long run.

It shows the relationship between inputs and outputs over an extended period. The change in the quantity of factors of production is called *scale*. All factors of production must be changed in the same proportion. For example, if all factors of production are doubled or tripled, large-scale production is achieved. Conversely, if all factors are reduced to half or one-third, production is carried out on a smaller scale. The resulting change in output is called *returns*.

Thus, the *law of returns to scale* explains changes in output due to changes in inputs over the long period.

Explanation of the Law

According to this law, when all inputs are increased in the same proportion, the output does not always increase in the same proportion. The change in output is classified into three stages:

1. Increasing Returns to Scale
2. Constant Returns to Scale
3. Diminishing Returns to Scale

1. Increasing Returns to Scale

If the proportionate increase in output is greater than the proportionate increase in inputs, it is termed *increasing returns to scale*. This means that when inputs are doubled, output increases by more than double.

Causes of Increasing Returns to Scale

- **Specialization or Division of Labor** – More workers lead to efficient production.
- **Indivisibility of Factors** – Some inputs (like machinery) cannot be divided; using them more efficiently increases output.
- **Dimensional Economics** – Larger production facilities reduce per-unit costs.
- **Volume Discounts** – Buying raw materials in bulk reduces costs.

2. Constant Returns to Scale

If the proportionate increase in output is equal to the proportionate increase in inputs, it is called *constant returns to scale*. This means that when inputs are doubled, output also doubles.

There are no specific causes for constant returns; it represents a balanced stage where inputs and outputs grow proportionally.

3. Diminishing Returns to Scale

If the proportionate increase in output is less than the proportionate increase in inputs, it is termed *diminishing returns to scale*. This means that when inputs are doubled, output increases by less than double.

Causes of Diminishing Returns to Scale

- **Management Problems** – Larger businesses become harder to coordinate.
- **Human Limitations** – Labour productivity may decline due to inefficiency at a larger scale.

Distinction between Returns to a Variable Factor and Returns to Scale

Scale of Operation	Inputs (Machines + Labor)	Output	Return to Scale
A	1 Machine + 2 Labor	100	-
B	2 Machines + 4 Labor	250	Increasing
C	4 Machines + 8 Labor	600	Increasing
D	8 Machines + 16 Labor	1200	Constant
E	16 Machines + 32 Labor	2400	Constant
F	32 Machines + 64 Labor	4000	Diminishing
G	64 Machines + 128 Labor	7000	Diminishing

Summary

1. **Increasing Returns to Scale** – Output increases more than proportionally to inputs.
2. **Constant Returns to Scale** – Output increases in the same proportion as inputs.
3. **Diminishing Returns to Scale** – Output increases less than proportionally to inputs.

Distinction between Returns to a Variable Factor and Returns to Scale

Returns to a Variable Factor	Returns to Scale
Operates in the short run and is related to the short-run production function.	Operates in the long run and is related to the long-run production function.
Only the quantity of the variable factor is varied.	All factor inputs are varied in the same proportion.
There is a change in the factor proportion.	There is no change in the factor ratio.
There is no change in the scale of production because all factor inputs are not changed.	There is a change in the scale of production because all factor inputs are varied in the same proportion.

Analytical Questions

Question 1

What is meant by a production function in the context of livestock farming?

Answer

A production function in animal farming expresses the relationship between physical inputs (like labour, feed, land) and physical outputs (like milk, eggs, or meat), given a certain level of technology. It shows how changing inputs affects output levels.

Question 2

What does the Law of Variable Proportions state?

Answer

The Law of Variable Proportions states that in the short run, as more units of a variable input (e.g., labour or feed) are added to a fixed input (e.g., land or infrastructure), total output first increases at an increasing rate, then at a decreasing rate, and finally starts declining.

Question 3

Why is Stage II of the Law of Variable Proportions considered the most efficient stage for farm operations?

Answer

Because in Stage II, total output continues to increase (though at a diminishing rate), and both Average Product (AP) and Marginal Product (MP) are positive. This is the stage where inputs are used most efficiently without causing stress or wastage.

Question 4

A dairy farm produces 150 liters of milk with 5 workers. What is the Average Product (AP)?

Answer

AP = TP/L = 150/5 = 30 liters per worker

Question 5

A poultry entrepreneur increases the number of workers from 4 to 5, and egg production rises from 200 to 230 eggs/day. What is the Marginal Product (MP)?

Answer

MP = ΔTP / ΔL = (230 - 200) / (5 - 4) = 30 eggs per worker

Question 6

In a veterinary clinic, hiring one more technician increases the number of treated animals from 40 to 50. What is the MP of the technician?

Answer

MP = 50 - 40 = 10 animals

Question 7

If additional feed increases milk yield initially but then leads to indigestion in animals, which stage is the farmer operating in?

Answer

This reflects Stage III (Negative Returns) where excessive input causes output to decline due to inefficiencies or stress on animals.

Question 10

A poultry farmer wants to add more workers. How can understanding the Law of Variable Proportion help in making this decision?

Answer

By analyzing where they are on the production curve. If in Stage I or II, adding labour can increase output. But in Stage III, adding labour would reduce efficiency and output. Thus, the farmer should aim to operate in Stage II.

Question 11

How can a dairy entrepreneur use MP and AP to decide on feeding levels for cows?

Answer

If MP of additional feed is positive but declining, the entrepreneur is in Stage II – optimal for profits. If MP becomes negative, overfeeding is causing health and productivity issues, suggesting a need to reduce feed quantity.

Question 12

What does it mean when MP = 0 and TPP is at its peak? Should inputs be increased further?

Answer

This is the maximum efficiency point; increasing inputs beyond this will push operations into Stage III, leading to reduced output. Inputs should not be increased further.

Case Studies

Stage 1 (Increasing Returns): Enhancing Dairy Output with Additional Labour

Question

You are managing a dairy farm with 10 cows and one worker, producing 100 litres of milk per day. Upon employing a second worker, the milk output increases to 130 litres per day. Explain why this occurs and suggest an appropriate course of action.

Answer

In Stage 1, additional labour results in a rapid increase in output due to improved efficiency—continue adding resources prudently.

Explanation: The presence of two workers allows for better task coordination, leading to a significant rise in milk production (increasing returns).

Strategy: Engage an additional worker to further enhance milk yield. Announce: "Collaboration enhances dairy output!"

Execution: Instruct the workers: "Coordinate efforts to maximize production," and monitor cow performance closely.

Outcome: Milk production increases further as additional labour optimizes resource use in the initial stage.

2. Stage 2 (Diminishing Returns): Optimizing Poultry Feed Application

Question

You oversee a poultry farm with 500 chickens producing 400 eggs daily using one bag of feed. Adding a second bag increases egg production to 450, but a third bag yields only 460 eggs. Analyze the situation and recommend a suitable approach.

Answer

In Stage 2, additional inputs yield progressively smaller gains—identify the optimal input level.

Explanation: The chickens' capacity to utilise extra feed diminishes, resulting in a reduced increase in egg output (diminishing returns).

Strategy: Maintain usage at two bags of feed. Communicate: "Balanced feeding ensures healthy poultry!"

Execution: Advise your team: "Two bags are sufficient—avoid excess," and observe egg production stability.

Outcome: Consistent egg output is achieved without wasteful expenditure on additional feed.

3. Stage 3 (Negative Returns): Addressing Overcrowding in Goat Farming

Question

You are responsible for a goat farm housing 20 goats in a limited shed, yielding 40 litres of milk daily. Introducing 5 additional goats reduces milk output to 35 litres. Assess the issue and propose a corrective measure.

Answer

In Stage 3, excessive inputs lead to a decline in output—reduce overcrowding to restore efficiency.

- **Explanation:** Overcrowding causes stress among goats, decreasing milk production (negative returns).
- **Strategy:** Relocate 5 goats to a separate area. State: "Comfortable goats produce more milk!"
- **Execution:** Direct your team: "Provide adequate space for better results," and arrange alternative shelter.
- **Outcome:** Milk production recovers as reduced crowding alleviates stress on the goats.

4. Women in Livestock (Stage 2): Training Female Dairy Workers

Question

You are training three women to milk 15 cows, producing 300 litres of milk daily. Adding a fourth woman increases output to 320 litres, though the gain is modest. Interpret this scenario and suggest an effective plan.

Answer

In Stage 2, additional labour contributes less to output—operate at an efficient level.

- **Explanation:** Four women improve production, but the cows' milking capacity limits further gains (diminishing returns).
- **Strategy:** Retain four workers without further additions. Declare: "An efficient team maximises milk yield!"
- **Execution:** Encourage the women: "Your current effort is ideal—maintain it!" and acknowledge their contribution.
- **Outcome:** Stable milk production is sustained with an effective workforce, avoiding inefficiency.

5. Social Media (Stage 1): Expanding Veterinary Outreach

Question

You are a veterinary professional promoting services through one social media advertisement per week, receiving 10 farmer inquiries. Increasing to two advertisements weekly raises inquiries to 15. Evaluate this development and recommend a subsequent step.

Answer

In Stage 1, additional efforts significantly enhance results—continue expanding outreach.

- **Explanation:** More advertisements reach a wider audience, increasing inquiries substantially (increasing returns).
- **Strategy:** Increase to three advertisements per week to attract more farmers. Promote: "Greater visibility, greater care!"
- **Execution:** Inform farmers online: "Contact us for expert veterinary support!" and monitor response rates.
- **Outcome:** Inquiries rise further as enhanced social media efforts yield greater engagement in the early stage.

Law of Variable Proportion (Short Run)

1. What is the Law of Variable Proportion?

Answer

It explains the change in output when one input (like labor or feed) is varied while keeping others (like land or infrastructure) constant. Initially, output increases at an increasing rate, then at a decreasing rate, and finally may decline.

2. What are the three stages of the Law of Variable Proportion?

Answer

Stage I: Increasing Returns

Stage II: Diminishing Returns (Optimal Stage)

Stage III: Negative Returns

3. Why is Stage II considered optimal for production?

Answer

Because in Stage II, although the marginal product is declining, it is still positive, and total output is maximized before inefficiencies set in.

4. Define Marginal Product with an example.

Answer

It is the additional output from one more unit of variable input.

Example: If adding 1 worker increases milk from 100L to 110L, MP = 10L.

5. In a poultry unit, what could be an example of entering Stage III of the law?

Answer

Overcrowding of birds beyond the optimal capacity in a poultry house leading to reduced growth and egg production.

6. What happens to Total Product (TP) when Marginal Product becomes zero?

Answer

Total Product reaches its maximum. This marks the end of Stage II.

Law of Returns to Scale (Long Run)

1. What is the Law of Returns to Scale?

Answer

It explains how output changes when all inputs are increased in the same proportion over the long run.

2. Name and define the three types of returns to scale.

Answer

Increasing Returns to Scale: Output increases more than proportionally to inputs.

Constant Returns to Scale: Output increases in the same proportion as inputs.

Diminishing Returns to Scale: Output increases less than proportionally to inputs.

3. Why do increasing returns to scale occur in large dairy or poultry farms?

Answer

Due to specialization, bulk purchasing, efficient machinery use, and economies of scale.

4. How can a veterinary entrepreneur experience diminishing returns to scale?

Answer

When rapid expansion leads to managerial inefficiencies, poor coordination, or underutilization of veterinary equipment or labor.

5. Differentiate between the Law of Variable Proportion and Returns to Scale

Feature	Returns to a Variable Factor	Returns to Scale
Time Frame	Short Run	Long Run
Inputs Changed	Only variable input	All inputs in same proportion
Factor Ratio	Changes	Remains Constant
Scale of Production	No change	Change in scale

6. If a farmer doubles his feed, land, and labour and milk output increases more than double, which stage is this?

Answer

This is increasing Returns to Scale.

7. What role does specialization play in increasing returns to scale?

Answer

Specialization improves efficiency, reduces wastage, and leads to more output from the same effort.

Law of Returns to Scale – Advanced Questions

1. A dairy entrepreneur triples inputs (land, feed, labor), but output only doubles. What kind of returns to scale is this?

Answer

Diminishing Returns to Scale – Output increases less than proportionately.

2. What kind of cost advantage is achieved when a poultry farmer gets feed at a lower price due to bulk purchasing?

Answer

Economy of Scale – Specifically, Purchasing Economies.

3. Which returns to scale is most desirable for business expansion?

Answer

Increasing Returns to Scale – It shows efficient and profitable growth.

4. Name two internal factors that lead to increasing returns to scale.

Answer

Specialization of labor and machines

Better utilization of fixed resources (like sheds, land, equipment)

5. What does "no change in factor ratio" mean in returns to scale?

Answer

It means all inputs are increased in the same proportion, keeping their ratio constant.

6. A veterinary clinic increases all staff and equipment by 100%, and services increase by only 60%. What is this an example of?

Answer

Diminishing Returns to Scale – Output increases less than inputs.

Law of Variable Proportion – Scenario-Based Questions

1. In a dairy farm, what happens if you keep increasing labor but don't expand milking machines or space?

Answer

You will enter Diminishing Returns – output per laborer will fall.

2. What's the marginal product if adding one more farmhand increases daily milk yield from 200 to 230 liters?

Answer

Marginal Product = 30 liters

3. How does the Law of Variable Proportion help in cost control?

Answer

It helps identify the most efficient level of input use, avoiding overuse and waste.

4. What marks the beginning of Stage III in the Law of Variable Proportion?

Answer

When Marginal Product becomes negative.

5. A poultry farmer adds more workers but observes bird mortality increasing due to poor coordination. Which stage is this?

Answer

Stage III – Negative Returns

Critical Thinking & Comparison Questions

1. Why can't the Law of Returns to Scale be applied in the short run?

Answer

Because in the short run, all inputs cannot be changed—some (like buildings, land) remain fixed.

2. What is the main assumption behind the Law of Returns to Scale?

Answer

All factors of production are variable and can be changed in the same proportion.

3. Why might returns to scale eventually diminish even in a well-managed poultry enterprise?

Answer

Because of management complexity, coordination difficulties, and resource constraints at very large scales.

4. What's the difference in focus between the two laws?

Law	**Focus**
Variable Proportion	Efficiency of a single input
Returns to Scale	Efficiency of all inputs combined

Analytical Questions

1. Increasing Returns to Scale: Expanding a Dairy Farm

Question 1

You operate a dairy farm with 1 machine and 2 workers, producing 100 litres of milk daily. By doubling your resources to 2 machines and 4 workers, output rises to 250 litres daily. Analyse why this occurs and recommend an appropriate strategy.

Answer

In Increasing Returns to Scale, output grows more than inputs—expand further to benefit.

- **Explanation:** Doubling inputs boosts efficiency through better machine use and worker teamwork, yielding more milk (increasing returns).
- **Strategy:** Triple resources to 3 machines and 6 workers. State: "Larger scale, greater milk!"
- **Execution:** Instruct your team: "Utilise additional resources effectively," and acquire more equipment.

- **Outcome:** Milk production increases significantly, leveraging specialization and scale advantages.

2. Constant Returns to Scale: Scaling a Poultry Business

Question

You manage a poultry farm with 4 machines and 8 workers, producing 600 eggs daily. Doubling to 8 machines and 16 workers results in 1200 eggs daily. Evaluate this situation and suggest a suitable course of action.

Answer

In Constant Returns to Scale, output matches input growth—maintain steady expansion.

- **Explanation:** Doubling resources doubles egg output, showing a balanced increase with no extra gain or loss (constant returns).
- **Strategy:** Continue scaling proportionally, such as to 12 machines and 24 workers. Announce: "Steady growth, steady eggs!"
- **Execution:** Advise your workers: "Keep operations consistent with more resources," and invest accordingly.
- **Outcome:** Egg production grows reliably in line with resources, ensuring stable operations.

3. Diminishing Returns to Scale: Managing a Veterinary Clinic

Question

You run a veterinary clinic with 16 machines and 32 workers, treating 2400 animals monthly. Doubling to 32 machines and 64 workers increases treatment to only 4000 animals. Assess the issue and propose a corrective measure.

Answer

In Diminishing Returns to Scale, output grows less than inputs—avoid over-expansion.

- **Explanation:** Doubling resources leads to coordination issues, so animal treatments rise less than expected (diminishing returns).
- **Strategy:** Scale back to 24 machines and 48 workers. Declare: "Efficient size, better care!"
- **Execution:** Direct your team: "Focus on manageable growth," and reduce excess equipment.
- **Outcome:** Treatment numbers improve relative to resources, avoiding management overload.

4. Women in Livestock (Increasing Returns): Growing a Women-Led Dairy Cooperative

Question

You support a women-led dairy cooperative with 1 machine and 2 women, producing 150 litres of milk daily. Doubling to 2 machines and 4 women raises output to 350 litres. Interpret this development and suggest a plan.

Answer

In Increasing Returns to Scale, output exceeds input growth—encourage further scaling.

- **Explanation:** More women and machines improve teamwork and efficiency, boosting milk more than double (increasing returns).
- **Strategy:** Expand to 3 machines and 6 women. Promote: "Women's teamwork grows milk!"
- **Execution:** Tell the women: "Add more hands and tools for bigger results," and secure resources.
- **Outcome:** Milk output rises further as women leverage scale benefits effectively.

5. Social Media (Constant Returns): Boosting Poultry Sales Online

Question

You promote poultry sales with 4 social media workers and 8 devices, selling 600 kg of chicken monthly. Doubling to 8 workers and 16 devices increases sales to 1200 kg. Examine this scenario and recommend a step forward.

Answer

In Constant Returns to Scale, output grows with inputs—keep scaling steadily.

- **Explanation:** Doubling workers and devices doubles sales, showing a proportional rise with no extra boost (constant returns).
- **Strategy:** Scale to 12 workers and 24 devices. Say: "More posts, more sales!"
- **Execution:** Instruct your team: "Maintain efforts with more tools," and expand online reach.
- **Outcome:** Chicken sales grow consistently, matching resource increases for reliable profits.

8

Factors of Production: Land, Labour, Capital & Entrepreneurship

The goods and services with the help of which the process of production is carried out, are called factors of production. Economists talk about **four main factors of production: land, labour, capital and entrepreneurship (or organization).** They are also called as the inputs of production. On the other hand, the goods produced with the help of these inputs, are called as the output.

1. Land

Land refers to all natural resources such as forests, water, climate, and soil. It provides space for livestock farms and raw materials for the dairy and meat industries.

Features of Land

1. **Gift of Nature** – Land and climatic conditions are naturally available. For example, the fertile plains of Punjab and Haryana are naturally suited for growing fodder crops like berseem and maize, which are essential for dairy farming. Similarly, the lush green pastures of Uttarakhand, Jammu & Kashmir and Himachal Pradesh provide an ideal environment for rearing sheep and goats.
2. **Limited in Supply** – Land is fixed, and certain resources like water bodies and fodder resources may deplete over time. Water scarcity in regions like Maharashtra has forced farmers to shift from water-intensive crops to drought-resistant fodder crops.
3. **Immobile Factor** – Land cannot be moved from one place to another, but its use can be altered. For instance, a farmer may convert land from wheat cultivation to fodder production for dairy animals.
4. **Diminishing Returns** – Excessive use of land without proper management may lead to reduced productivity. For example, continuous cultivation of fodder crops without crop rotation or soil enrichment has resulted in declining yields, forcing farmers to invest in expensive fertilizers.

5. **Differences in Fertility** – Some lands are more productive than others. For example, low-fertility soils in high-altitude regions make it difficult to grow certain fodder crops.
6. **Passivity** – Land is a passive factor of production. It does not actively participate in production but is acted upon by labour and machinery. For instance, the barren lands of Kutch in Gujarat were transformed into productive grazing lands through community-led afforestation and water conservation initiatives.

2. Labour

Labour refers to any form of human effort, physical or mental, undertaken to earn economic rewards. In economics, labour includes only human work, excluding tasks performed by animals or machines. In animal husbandry, labour is essential for tasks like milking, feeding, and managing livestock.

Features of Labour

1. **Inseparable from the Labourer** – Unlike land and capital, labour cannot be separated from the person performing it.
2. **Perishable** – If labour is not utilized on a given day, it is lost forever. For example, if a dairy worker skips milking a cow, the lost milk cannot be recovered.
3. **Means and End of Production** – Labour not only helps in wealth production but is also essential for satisfying human needs. For example, women in rural Rajasthan who work in dairy cooperatives not only contribute to milk production but also earn income to support their families.
4. **Investment in Labour** – Labour can be enhanced through education, skill development, and physical well-being, often referred to as **human capital**. For example, the government has introduced training programs for livestock farmers on modern dairy practices, leading to increased milk production and better animal health management.

3. Capital

Capital refers to man-made resources like machinery, tools, buildings, and money used in production. It enhances the efficiency and productivity of land and labour.

Features of Capital

1. **Supplies Tools and Machines:** Capital provides tools and machines that improve productivity. For example, chaff cutters and milking machines improve efficiency in dairy farms.

2. **Improves Productivity of Labour:** Better tools and equipment enhance the efficiency of labour. For example, automatic feeding systems in poultry farms reduce manual effort and increase production.
3. **Supplies Raw Materials:** Capital ensures a continuous supply of raw materials like feed, fodder, and medicines. For example, feed supplements and vaccines are essential for maintaining milk production in dairy farms.
4. **Generates Employment**: Capital investment leads to job creation. For example, establishing a large dairy processing unit creates employment for farm workers, veterinarians, and transporters.
5. **Provides Transport Facilities:** Capital in the form of infrastructure (roads, railways) helps transport raw materials and finished goods. For example, the Pradhan Mantri Gram Sadak Yojana has improved access to markets for livestock farmers in remote areas.
6. **Payments to Factors**: Entrepreneurs use capital to pay wages and other expenses. For example, a dairy farmer pays workers in advance before selling milk in the market.

Types of Capital

Capital refers to man-made resources used in production.

1. Capital supplies tools and machines. It is classified into several types:

1. Fixed Capital & Working Capital

i. **Fixed Capital** –Durable and long-lasting assets used repeatedly in production, such as buildings, machinery, and tools. Examples in animal husbandry Durable assets like dairy farm buildings, milking machines, and tractors. For example, a dairy cooperative in Gujarat invested in a bulk milk cooler to preserve milk quality.

ii. **Working Capital** – Used up in production and not reusable, such as feed, fodder, and fuel. For instance, a poultry farmer purchases feed and medicines on a monthly basis.

2. Individual Capital & Social Capital

i. **Individual Capital** – Assets owned privately by individuals, such as personal equipment and machinery. Privately owned assets like a farmer's personal tractor or milking equipment.

ii. **Social Capital** – Infrastructure that benefits society, such as public roads and bridges. Public infrastructure like veterinary hospitals and rural roads. For example, the Pradhan Mantri Gram Sadak Yojana has improved access to markets for livestock farmers in remote areas.

3. Material Capital & Personal Capital

i. **Material Capital** – Tangible assets that can be bought or sold, such as land and machinery, livestock sheds and milking machines.

ii. **Personal Capital** – Intangible qualities such as intelligence, skills, and work ethic that contribute to productivity. Example include intangible qualities like a farmer's knowledge of animal nutrition or disease management.

> **Understanding Four Factors of Production in Dairy Farming**
>
> **Examples of Inputs/Factors of Production:**
>
> i. Land: Pastureland and fields for growing fodder crops like berseem and maize.
>
> ii. Labour: Workers for milking, feeding, and managing cattle.
>
> iii. Capital: Milking machines, storage tanks, and veterinary equipment.
>
> iv. Entrepreneurship: A dairy cooperative organizing farmers, managing supply chains, and marketing milk to urban consumers.
>
> **Outputs**
>
> i. Milk, butter, cheese, and other dairy products.
>
> ii. Employment opportunities and income for rural communities.

Money Capital & Real Capital

i. **Money Capital** – Financial resources available for investment and business expansion. For example, loans or savings used to invest in livestock farming.

ii. **Real Capital** – Physical assets like dairy machines, equipment, and tools used in production.

4. Entrepreneur

An entrepreneur organizes and manages production by combining land, labour, and capital.

Roles of an Entrepreneur

1. **Decision Making** – Determines production size and marketing strategies. For instance, a poultry farm owner chooses between broiler and layer farming based on market demand.
2. **Choosing Technology** – Selects appropriate production methods and tools. In Punjab, dairy farmers have started using automated milking machines to increase efficiency and reduce labour costs.
3. **Innovation** – Introduces new ideas, techniques, and products. For instance, farmers in Maharashtra have adopted hydroponic fodder cultivation, which uses less water and space compared to traditional methods, to feed dairy cattle.

4. **Paying Rewards to Factors of Production** – Entrepreneurs compensate labour, capital, and landowners for their contributions. For example, owner/group of owners of a milk processing plant pays wages to workers, rent to landowners, and interest to lenders.
5. **Bearing Profit/Loss Risks** – Entrepreneurs bear the financial risks of business operations. For example, a milk processing plant owner pays wages to workers but bears the loss if milk prices fall. Further, during the COVID-19 pandemic, many poultry farmers in India faced losses due to a sudden drop in demand, but they also adapted by selling directly to consumers through online platforms.

Capitalist vs. Entrepreneur

i. **A Capitalist** is a person who owns capital, invests it, and earns interest. Regardless of profit or loss, the capitalist receives a fixed return. For example, a venture capitalist provides capital to dairy entrepreneurs at a fixed interest rate.

ii. An **Entrepreneur** takes business risks and is responsible for profits and losses. For instance, a dairy entrepreneur invests in a high-tech feed unit and bears the risk of fluctuating feed demand and prices.

iii. In practice, a person may be both a capitalist and an entrepreneur.

CASE STUDY-Based Questions and Answers

CASE STUDY 1: Decision-Making in Poultry Farming

Scenario

Arun, a young entrepreneur, wants to start a poultry farm in Tamil Nadu. He is confused between broiler farming (for meat production) and layer farming (for egg production). After researching, he finds that local market demand for eggs is high due to a rise in health-conscious consumers.

Question

How did Arun's decision-making as an entrepreneur influence his poultry business, and why is market demand an essential factor?

Answer

- Arun's **decision-making** was based on **analyzing market demand**, a key trait of a successful entrepreneur.
- Since **egg consumption** was rising, he **chose layer farming**, ensuring steady demand and profits.
- This case highlights how **understanding market trends** helps entrepreneurs make **informed business choices**.

CASE STUDY 2: Choosing Technology in Dairy Farming

Scenario

A dairy farmer in Punjab was struggling with high labour costs for milking his 30 cows. To reduce dependency on labour, he invested in an automated milking machine. After installation, he noticed that the milking process became faster, and hygiene improved, leading to better milk quality and higher profits.

Question

Why is choosing the right technology important for a dairy entrepreneur, and how did automation help this farmer?

Answer

- **Choosing technology** is vital as it **enhances efficiency, reduces costs, and improves productivity**.
- The **automated milking machine** helped the farmer by:
- **Reducing dependency on labour**, leading to cost savings.
- **Improving milk hygiene**, leading to **higher market value**.
- **Saving time**, allowing the farmer to focus on other aspects of the business.
- This case highlights how **technological innovation** can help **entrepreneurs stay competitive** in the dairy industry.

CASE STUDY 3: Innovation in Fodder Cultivation

Scenario

A group of dairy farmers in Maharashtra faced fodder shortages due to irregular rainfall. To solve this problem, they adopted hydroponic fodder cultivation, which grows fodder using minimal water and no soil. This allowed them to provide a steady supply of green fodder, improving cattle health and milk yield.

Question

How does innovation play a role in entrepreneurial success, and why was hydroponic fodder a good solution?

Answer

- **Innovation** is crucial for entrepreneurs to **overcome challenges** and **increase efficiency**.
- **Hydroponic fodder cultivation** was beneficial because:

  - It **required less water**, making it ideal for drought-prone areas.
  - It **ensured a regular supply of green fodder**, leading to **better cattle health**.
  - It **increased milk production**, improving farmers' profits.
- This case shows that **innovative approaches** can help **agri-entrepreneurs** tackle industry challenges.

CASE STUDY 4: Bearing Profit and Loss Risks in the Poultry Industry

Scenario

During the COVID-19 pandemic, poultry farmers in India suffered huge losses due to a sudden drop in demand. However, Ramesh, a poultry entrepreneur, quickly adapted by selling his eggs and chicken directly to consumers via online platforms. This helped him recover losses and even expand his customer base.

Question

How do entrepreneurs bear risks, and what strategy did Ramesh use to survive during the crisis?

Answer

- Entrepreneurs must **accept business risks** and find **solutions to challenges**.
- Ramesh **bore the loss initially** but recovered by:
  - **Using online sales channels** to reach consumers directly.
  - **Eliminating middlemen**, ensuring better profits.
  - **Providing home delivery**, increasing customer convenience.
- This case highlights that **adaptability and quick decision-making** are essential for **entrepreneurs facing market fluctuations**.

CASE STUDY 5: Capitalist vs. Entrepreneur in Dairy Processing

Scenario

A venture capitalist invested ₹ 50 lakhs in a milk processing plant. The plant's owner, Priya, used the funds to set up modern pasteurization and packaging units. While the capitalist earned a fixed return on investment, Priya took the business risk and earned profits by selling packaged milk.

Question

How does this scenario illustrate the difference between a capitalist and an entrepreneur?

Answer

- The **venture capitalist** is an **investor** who provides **financial support** but does not manage the business. They **earn interest** regardless of the plant's performance.
- Priya, the **entrepreneur**, **manages operations**, **takes risks**, and **bears profits or losses**.
- **Key Difference**
    - **Capitalists** earn fixed returns.
    - **Entrepreneurs** earn profits but also face business risks.
- This case emphasizes that while **capitalists provide funding, entrepreneurs drive business success**.

CASE STUDY 6: Land Utilization in Dairy Farming

Scenario

Ramesh, a dairy farmer in Punjab, has been growing wheat on his 5-acre land for years. Due to increasing demand for milk, he is considering converting part of his land into a fodder farm to support his growing herd of cattle. However, he is worried about soil fertility and long-term sustainability.

Questions

1. *How does the concept of* ***land as a factor of production*** *apply to Ramesh's situation?*
2. *What steps can Ramesh take to* ***maintain soil fertility*** *while transitioning to fodder crops?*
3. *How does* ***diminishing returns*** *impact his decision, and how can he mitigate this risk?*

Answers

1. Land is a **gift of nature** and is **immobile**, meaning Ramesh cannot move his farm but can alter its use. By shifting from wheat cultivation to fodder production, he is optimizing his **land resources** to support his dairy business.
2. Ramesh can practice **crop rotation**, use **organic manure** from his dairy waste, and adopt **soil enrichment techniques** such as composting to maintain soil fertility.
3. Excessive fodder cultivation without soil management can lead to **diminishing returns**. To mitigate this, Ramesh should implement

sustainable farming practices, such as **rotational grazing**, **green manure application**, and **water-efficient irrigation systems**.

CASE STUDY 7: Land Fertility Issues in Sheep Rearing

Scenario

Mohit, a sheep farmer in Himachal Pradesh, struggles with low-fertility soil in high-altitude areas, limiting fodder crop growth. He is considering shifting to a pasture-based system for his livestock.

Questions

1. *How does **land fertility variation** affect Mohit's livestock business?*
2. *What **alternative fodder solutions** can he explore to sustain his sheep farming?*
3. *How does **land passivity** influence his production process, and how can he improve it?*

Answers

1. Poor **soil fertility** leads to **low-quality pasture**, affecting sheep nutrition and productivity.
2. He can use **high-altitude fodder crops**, introduce **silvopastoral systems (trees + grass)**, and practice **rotational grazing** to improve pasture availability.
3. Land is **passive** and requires **active management** through **irrigation**, **fertilization**, and **community-driven afforestation** efforts to enhance grazing areas.

CASE STUDY 8: Veterinary Start-up for Rural Farmers

Question

Dr. Arjun, a veterinarian, wants to set up a mobile veterinary clinic to serve rural dairy and poultry farmers in his region. He has expertise (human capital) but lacks funds for a vehicle, medicines, and equipment. What factors of production should he consider, and how can he secure the necessary capital?

Answer

Dr. Arjun should consider the following factors:

- **Land:** Operating in rural areas, he does not need fixed land but requires routes and access to farms.
- **Labour:** He may need assistants for record-keeping and animal handling.

- **Capital:** A vehicle, medical equipment, and vaccines require financial investment.
- **Entrepreneurship:** Managing operations, marketing services, and ensuring sustainability are his key roles.

To secure capital, he can

1. **Seek Government Grants** – Programs like the Rashtriya Gokul Mission may provide financial aid.
2. **Crowdfunding** – He can raise funds through online platforms or local dairy cooperatives.
3. **Microfinance Loans** – Small business loans from rural banks or NGOs can help him acquire essential resources.
4. **Collaborations with Dairy Cooperatives** – Partnering with milk unions can provide financial backing and a steady customer base.

With a strategic approach, Dr. Arjun can establish a successful mobile veterinary service in rural areas.

CASE STUDY 9: Labour Shortage in a Dairy Farm

Scenario

A dairy farm in Rajasthan with 50 cows is facing a labour shortage as several workers have migrated to cities for better job opportunities. The remaining workers are struggling to complete daily tasks like milking, feeding, and cleaning. The farm owner, Ramesh, is considering investing in automated milking machines but is unsure if this will be cost-effective.

Question

What are the possible solutions Ramesh can explore to address the labour shortage while maintaining milk production efficiency?

Answer

- **Invest in Automation:** Purchasing automated milking machines can reduce dependence on manual labour, ensuring timely milking and maintaining milk yield.
- **Training & Upskilling Existing Labour:** Training the remaining workers on modern dairy practices can help improve efficiency.
- **Attract Local Labour:** Offering better wages, incentives, and improved working conditions can help retain and attract local workers.
- **Flexible Work Schedules:** Implementing rotational shifts may help distribute workload among the remaining workers.

CASE STUDY 10: Perishable Nature of Labour in Poultry Farming

Scenario

A poultry farm in Tamil Nadu has 5,000 broiler birds. The owner, Priya, relies on daily manual feeding, cleaning, and vaccination by farmworkers. One day, a sudden worker strike disrupts the farm operations, delaying feeding and cleaning. As a result, some birds develop health issues, leading to a decline in meat quality.

Question

How does this situation highlight the perishable nature of labour? What steps can Priya take to prevent such issues in the future?

Answer

- Labour is perishable because if not used on a given day, it cannot be stored or recovered. The missed feeding and cleaning led to lower bird health, impacting meat quality and profitability.
- **Preventive Measures:**
  i. **Cross-training workers** to handle multiple tasks so that farm operations don't halt if a few workers are absent.
  ii. **Introducing automation** like automatic feeders and water systems to reduce dependency on manual labour.
  iii. **Maintaining a backup workforce** to step in during emergencies.
  iv. **Ensuring good worker relations** by addressing grievances to prevent strikes.

CASE STUDY 11: Women Empowerment in Dairy Cooperatives

Scenario

A dairy cooperative in Gujarat trains rural women in milk production and quality management. Many of these women, previously unemployed, now earn a stable income through dairy farming. Some have also started small-scale milk processing units to make paneer and ghee.

Question

How does this case demonstrate the role of labour as both a means and an end of production?

Answer

- **Labour as a Means of Production:** The women's work in dairy farming contributes to wealth generation by increasing milk production and supply.

- **Labour as an End of Production:** The women themselves benefit from their work by gaining income, improving their standard of living, and achieving financial independence.
- This example also highlights **investment in labour** through skill development, showing how training enhances productivity and economic empowerment.

CASE STUDY 12: Investment in Labour for Veterinary Services

Scenario

Dr. Anil, a young veterinarian, notices that many livestock farmers in Himachal Pradesh lack knowledge about disease prevention and proper feeding. He decides to conduct training sessions and workshops for farmers, teaching them about vaccination, deworming, and balanced diets. Over time, farmers report healthier livestock and increased milk production.

Question

How does investment in labour contribute to improved veterinary services and livestock management?

Answer

- Investing in **education and skill development** improves farmers' ability to manage livestock efficiently.
- Knowledge of **disease prevention and proper feeding** reduces veterinary costs and increases productivity.
- Trained farmers act as **local resource persons**, spreading veterinary knowledge within their communities, creating a sustainable impact.
- This also demonstrates **human capital formation**, where investing in training leads to long-term benefits for both farmers and veterinarians.

CASE STUDY 13. Inseparable from the Labourer: Keeping Dairy Workers Ready

Question

You have 2 workers milking 20 cows (500L milk/month at ₹50/L), paid ₹6,000/month. One worker gets sick, and milk drops to 400L. How can you keep work going since labour is tied to the worker?

Answer

Labour sticks with the person—make sure someone's always there.

- **Strategy:** Hire a backup worker for ₹2,000/month to keep milk at 500L. Say: "No milk lost!"

- **Execution:** Find a local helper fast (₹200 training cost). Give the sick worker ₹500 for medicine to come back soon. Tell buyers: "Milk's always ready—₹50/L."
- **Outcome:** You sell 500L (₹25,000), spend ₹8,200 (₹6,000 + ₹2,000 + ₹200), earn ₹16,800 vs. ₹14,000 (400L), keeping work steady.

CASE STUDY 14. Perishable: Saving Poultry Eggs Daily

Question

Your 1 worker (₹3,000/month) collects 800 eggs/day from 1,000 chickens (₹4,800/day at ₹6/egg). They miss a day, losing 800 eggs. How can you stop losing eggs since labour can't be saved?

Answer

Labour not used is gone—make sure it's there every day.

- **Strategy:** Pay a friend ₹300/day to collect eggs when your worker's off, keeping 800 eggs/day. Say: "Eggs every day!"
- **Execution:** Ask a neighbor to help 5 days/year (₹1,500 total). Tell buyers: "Fresh eggs always—₹6 each."
- **Outcome:** You sell ₹1,44,000/month (30 x ₹4,800), spend ₹4,500 (₹3,000 + ₹1,500), earn ₹1,39,500 vs. ₹1,34,700 (29 days), saving eggs daily.

CASE STUDY 15: Means and End of Production: Helping Dairy Workers Thrive

Question

Your 3 workers (₹9,000/month) make 600L milk/month (₹30,000 at ₹50/L). They're tired and unhappy, dropping to 500L. How can you use labour to make milk and support them?

Answer

Labour makes money and meets needs—keep workers happy.

- **Strategy:** Raise pay to ₹10,500/month to get 650L. Say: "Better pay, more milk!"
- **Execution:** Use extra milk money (₹2,500) to add ₹500/worker. Tell them: "You win, we win—₹50/L milk."
- **Outcome:** You sell 650L (₹32,500), spend ₹10,500, earn ₹22,000 vs. ₹16,000 (500L), boosting milk and worker lives.

CASE STUDY 16: Investment in Labour: Teaching Vet Helpers

Question

Your 1 helper (₹5,000/month) checks 30 animals/month at ₹400/visit. They can't do shots, missing 10 more jobs. How can you train them to grow your vet work?

Answer

Training makes labour better—teach new skills.

- **Strategy:** Spend ₹2,000 to train them for shots, aiming for 40 visits at ₹450/visit. Say: "More help, better care!"
- **Execution:** Join a free vet class, buy a shot kit (₹2,000). Tell farmers: "Full care now—₹450/visit."
- **Outcome:** You earn ₹18,000 (40 x ₹450), spend ₹7,000 (₹5,000 + ₹2,000), profit ₹11,000 vs. ₹7,000, growing with skilled help.

CASE STUDY 17. Combined Features: Growing Poultry Meat Work

Question

Your 2 workers (₹6,000/month) cut 500 kg chicken/month (₹1,00,000 at ₹200/kg). You want 600 kg, but they're slow and waste meat. How can you use labour's traits to get more?

Answer

Labour's tied to people, can't wait, and can improve—fix all three.

- **Strategy:** Train 1 worker (₹2,000) to cut faster, add a helper (₹2,000/month) for 600 kg. Keep ₹200/kg. Say: "More meat, no waste!"
- **Execution:** Teach cutting in 2 days (₹2,000), hire help for busy days (inseparability, perishability). Tell buyers: "Fresh meat daily—₹200/kg."
- **Outcome:** You sell 600 kg (₹1,20,000), spend ₹10,000 (₹6,000 + ₹2,000 + ₹2,000), earn ₹1,10,000 vs. ₹94,000, using labour smartly.

CASE STUDY 18: Fixed vs. Working Capital in a Dairy Farm

Scenario

Rahul owns a dairy farm in Punjab with 20 cows. He recently invested in a bulk milk cooler (BMC) to preserve milk quality before sending it to the market. However, he is struggling to cover the cost of daily feed and veterinary care for his animals.

Question

How does Rahul's investment in the bulk milk cooler represent fixed capital, and why is his struggle with feed and veterinary care related to working capital?

Answer

- **Fixed Capital:** The **bulk milk cooler** is a **long-term, durable asset** that will be used repeatedly to store milk, making it a **fixed capital investment**.
- **Working Capital:** Feed and veterinary care are **recurring expenses** that get **used up** in daily production and need to be **replenished regularly**, which classifies them as **working capital**.
- **Solution:** Rahul should **balance his capital investments**, ensuring that he reserves enough funds for **working capital** to sustain daily operations.

CASE STUDY 19: Impact of Social Capital on Dairy Business Expansion

Scenario

A dairy cooperative in Himachal Pradesh struggled to reach markets due to poor road conditions. However, after the Pradhan Mantri Gram Sadak Yojana improved rural roads, they expanded their business, increasing their milk supply to urban areas.

Question

How does the development of rural roads represent an investment in social capital, and how did it benefit the dairy cooperative?

Answer

- **Social Capital: Infrastructure improvements**, like better roads, **benefit the entire society**, making them a form of **social capital** rather than individual property.
- **Benefits to Dairy Cooperative:**
  - Easier and **faster transportation** of milk to markets, reducing spoilage.
  - **Lower transportation costs**, increasing profits.
  - **Increased farmer participation** in dairy farming due to improved market access.
- This highlights how **public infrastructure investment** can boost **entrepreneurial opportunities** in the dairy sector.

CASE STUDY 20: Money Capital vs. Real Capital in Poultry Farming

Scenario

Amit, a poultry farmer in Tamil Nadu, took a bank loan of ₹5 lakhs to expand his farm. He used ₹3 lakhs to buy automatic feeders and temperature control systems, while ₹2 lakhs were kept as emergency funds for feed purchases and unexpected veterinary expenses.

Question

How do Amit's investments represent money capital and real capital?

Answer

- **Money Capital:** The **₹5 lakh loan** is **money capital** as it represents **financial resources available for investment**.
- **Real Capital:** The **automatic feeders and temperature control systems** are **real capital** because they are **physical assets used in production**.
- **Importance:** A well-planned division of funds between **long-term assets (real capital)** and **operational needs (working capital)** is crucial for a **sustainable poultry business**.

CASE STUDY 21: Investment in Personal Capital for Veterinary Entrepreneurs

Scenario

Dr. Meera, a veterinarian, noticed a gap in rural veterinary services in Uttarakhand. She attended specialized training on modern livestock disease management and started her own mobile veterinary service. Farmers now rely on her expertise for disease prevention and livestock health management.

Question

How does Dr. Meera's training and expertise represent an investment in personal capital, and how does it benefit livestock farmers?

Answer

- **Personal Capital:** Dr. Meera's **knowledge and skills** are a form of **personal capital**, as they are **intangible assets** that enhance her ability to provide **veterinary services**.
- **Benefits to Farmers:**
  - i **Access to expert veterinary care**, reducing livestock mortality.
  - ii **Increased productivity** as healthier animals produce more milk and meat.

iii **Growth of her veterinary business**, benefiting both **her income** and the **rural economy**.

- This case highlights the **importance of education and skill development** in the **veterinary and animal husbandry sectors**.

CASE STUDY 22. Supplies Tools and Machines: Boosting Dairy Milk Output

Question

You're a dairy farmer with 10 cows making 250L milk/month (₹12,500 at ₹50/L). Milking by hand is slow. How can tools from capital help you get more milk?

Answer

Capital gives tools to work faster—use machines.

- **Strategy:** Buy a ₹20,000 milking machine (fixed capital) to milk faster, aiming for 300L/month. Keep ₹50/L price.
- **Execution:** Say: "Quick milk, same taste!" Pay ₹5,000 now, ₹15,000 later (loan). Milk 10 cows in half the time.
- **Outcome:** You sell 300L (₹15,000), spend ₹7,000 (feed, labor), earn ₹8,000 vs. ₹5,500, as tools raise output.

CASE STUDY 23. Improves Productivity of Labour: Helping Poultry Workers

Question

Your 2 workers (₹6,000/month) feed 1,000 chickens by hand, producing 800 eggs/day (₹4,800/day at ₹6/egg). It's hard work. How can capital make their job easier?

Answer

Capital boosts worker speed—add equipment.

- **Strategy:** Get an automatic feeder (₹10,000, fixed capital) for 900 eggs/day. Keep ₹6/egg.
- **Execution:** Say: "Less work, more eggs!" Pay ₹2,000 down, rest over time. Workers finish faster, happier.
- **Outcome:** You sell ₹5,400/day (900 x ₹6), ₹1,62,000/month, spend ₹7,000 (₹6,000 + ₹1,000 depreciation), earn ₹1,55,000 vs. ₹1,38,000, as capital helps labour.

CASE STUDY 24. Supplies Raw Materials: Keeping Vet Clinic Stocked

Question

You run a vet clinic treating 30 animals/month (₹400/visit, ₹12,000). You run out of medicines often, losing 5 visits. How can capital keep supplies ready?

Answer

Capital buys raw materials—stock up.

- **Strategy:** Spend ₹5,000/month on extra medicines (working capital) for 35 visits. Raise to ₹450/visit.
- **Execution:** Say: "Care always ready—₹450!" Buy bulk vaccines (₹4,000), bandages (₹1,000). Tell farmers: "No delays."
- **Outcome:** You earn ₹15,750 (35 x ₹450), spend ₹10,000 (₹5,000 staff + ₹5,000 supplies), profit ₹5,750 vs. ₹2,000, as capital ensures supplies.

CASE STUDY 25.Capital Generates Employment: Growing Dairy Jobs

Question

You make 500L milk/month (₹25,000 at ₹50/L) with 2 workers (₹6,000/ month). You want to add butter and hire more people. How can capital create jobs?

Answer

Capital investments make jobs—expand with it.

- **Strategy:** Buy a ₹30,000 butter churner (fixed capital), hire 1 worker (₹3,000/month) for 100 kg butter (₹40,000 at ₹400/kg).
- **Execution:** Say: "Milk and butter, more help!" Pay₹10,000 now, rest later. Sell butter to shops.
- **Outcome:** Revenue ₹65,000 (₹25,000 milk + ₹40,000 butter), costs ₹19,000 (₹9,000 labour + ₹10,000 other), profit ₹46,000 vs. ₹19,000, adding jobs with capital.

CASE STUDY 26. Capital Provides transport facilities: moving poultry eggs

Question

You sell 1,000 eggs/day (₹6,000 at ₹6/egg) from a remote farm, but bad roads lose you 200 eggs/day. How can capital fix transport to sell more?

Answer

Capital builds transport—get goods moving.

- **Strategy:** Buy a ₹50,000 bike (fixed capital) to deliver 1,200 eggs/day. Keep ₹6/egg.
- **Execution:** Say: "Eggs on time!" Pay ₹10,000 down, ₹40,000 loan (₹1,000/month cost). Reach 5 new buyers.
- **Outcome:** Revenue ₹7,200/day (1,200 x ₹6), ₹2,16,000/month, costs ₹11,000 (₹6,000 labour + ₹5,000 other), profit ₹2,05,000 vs. ₹1,74,000, as transport capital grows sales.

References

Bardhan, D. (2018). Textbook on Livestock Economics, Marketing & Business Management. New India Publishing Agency. ISBN: 9789381226315.

FAO (Food and Agriculture Organization). (2018). The State of Food and Agriculture: Livestock Contributions. Rome: FAO.

Gangadhar, K. S., & Satyanarayan, K. (2022). Livestock Economics, Marketing, Entrepreneurship, Business Management & Accountancy (2nd fully revised & enlarged ed.). New Delhi: New India Publishing Agency.

Herrero, M., et al. (2013). "Biomass Use, Production, Feed Efficiencies, and Greenhouse Gas Emissions from Global Livestock Systems." Proceedings of the National Academy of Sciences, 110(52), 20888–20893.

ILRI (International Livestock Research Institute). (2020). Livestock and Livelihoods: Economic Impacts. Nairobi: ILRI.

Keynes, J. M. (1936). The General Theory of Employment, Interest, and Money. London: Macmillan.

Marshall, A. (1890). Principles of Economics. London: Macmillan.

Robbins, L. (1932). An Essay on the Nature and Significance of Economic Science. London: Macmillan.

Samuelson, P. A. (1948). Economics: An Introductory Analysis. New York: McGraw-Hill.

Smith, A. (1776). An Inquiry into the Nature and Causes of the Wealth of Nations. London: W. Strahan & T. Cadell.

Subba Reddy, S., Raghu Ram, P., Neelakanta Sastry, T. V., & Bhavani Devi, I. (2016). Agricultural Economics (2nd ed.). Kochi: CBS Publishers; New Delhi: Oxford and IBH Publishing. ISBN: 9788120417861.

The Institute of Cost Accountants of India (ICAI). (2014). Fundamentals of Economics and Management: Study Notes (Foundation Paper - 1) (2nd ed.). Kolkata: Directorate of Studies, The Institute of Cost Accountants of India.

Index

About the Editor

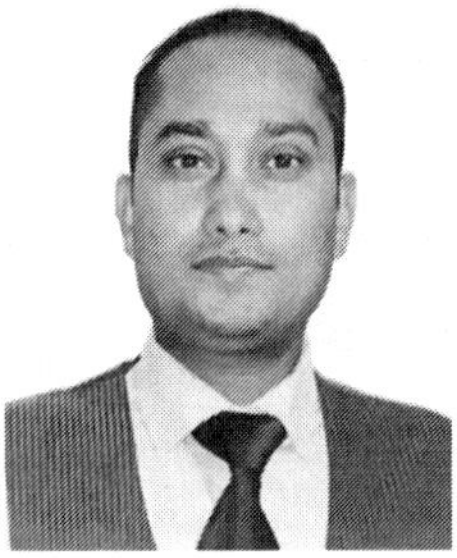

Dr. Avinash Kumar, Assistant Professor-cum-Junior Scientist, Department of Agricultural Economics, Bihar Agricultural College, Sabour, Bhagalpur, Bihar, India. He is a dedicated academician and accomplished editor with over six years of professional experience in agricultural economics and textbook development. He is currently serving as an Assistant Professor-cum-Junior Scientist at the Department of Agricultural Economics, Bihar Agricultural College, Sabour—one of the oldest agricultural colleges in India—since September 2023.Dr. Kumar earned his Ph.D. in Agricultural Economics from CSK Himachal Pradesh Krishi Vishvavidyalaya (CSK HPKV), Palampur in 2022. Since September 2023, he has been serving at Bihar Agricultural College, Sabour. He holds a Ph.D. in Agricultural Economics from CSK HPKV, Palampur (2022), an M.Sc. from GBPUAT, Pantnagar (2015), and a B.Sc. in Horticulture from UHS, Bagalkot (2012). He has qualified NET in Agricultural Economics (UGC and ICAR) and received ICAR fellowships including NTS, JRF, and SRF. Dr. Kumar previously taught at Lovely Professional University (2019–2023), handling courses like Econometrics and Agricultural Finance while contributing to textbook editing. He has authored 24 publications, including 17 research papers, 3 book chapters, and holds 3 patents and 2 copyrights. He has guided 11 M.Sc. students as a minor advisor.

His research interests include econometrics, production economics, and agricultural marketing, with strong skills in MS Office, LaTeX, SPSS, R, and Python.